ECHINACEA

NATURE'S REMEDIES

ECHINACEA

The Plant that Boosts Your Immune System

Douglas Schar

SOUVENIR PRESS

First published 1999 by
Souvenir Press Ltd,
43 Great Russell Street, London WC1B 3PA

ISBN 0 285 63488 7

Typeset by Rowland Phototypesetting Ltd,
Bury St Edmunds, Suffolk

Printed in Great Britain by
The Guernsey Press Company Ltd,
Guernsey, Channel Islands

Acknowledgements

This study of Echinacea is dedicated to a number of very special people without whose assistance and support it would not have become a reality. Working as a professional in the field of herbal medicine is not easy in a world that does not accept it, and those of us who do lean heavily on those around us.

To Paul Johnson, who has put up with my ups and downs for some time now and only complains occasionally.

To Dawn Clarke, who worked hard with me, and sacrificed her eyesight, to complete this book.

To Sarah O'Donnell, alternative medicine editor at *Prevention* magazine. Sarah has been a source of inspiration and support from the first time we met. She has reaffirmed my faith in humanity.

To my father, who taught me to think beyond the obvious, to see opportunities where there appear to be none, and to question everything.

To my mother, who always encouraged and indulged me.

To the members of the Herbalists of Columbia Road Think-Tank, Denise Turner, Roz Christenson and Stuart FitzSimmons.

To Adrian Thornton for being so supportive of the Herbalists on Columbia Road—HCR—and believing in us before there was a reason to do so.

That is just the beginning of the list of people who need to be thanked for their contribution to this book, and indeed to my career in herbal medicine.

Note to Readers

The aim of this book is to provide information on the uses of Echinacea in the treatment of relevant diseases. Although every care has been taken to ensure that the advice is accurate and practical, it is not intended to be a guide to self-diagnosis and self-treatment. Where health is concerned—and in particular a serious problem of any kind—it must be stressed that there is no substitute for seeking advice from a qualified medical practitioner. All persistent symptoms, of whatever nature, may have underlying causes that need, and should not be treated without, professional elucidation and evaluation.

It is therefore very important, if you are considering trying Echinacea, to consult your practitioner first, and if you are already taking any prescribed medication, do not stop it.

The Publisher makes no representation, express or implied, with regard to the accuracy of the information contained in this book, and legal responsibility or liability cannot be accepted by the Author or the Publisher for any errors or omissions that may be made or for any loss, damage, injury or problems suffered or in any way arising from following the advice offered in these pages.

Contents

Introduction

365,000,000 AMERICAN DOLLARS

You may think that figure represents the annual budget for a major government ministry. In fact, it is the amount of money Americans spent on Echinacea in 1997. It is hard to estimate how much more was spent in Europe on this medicinal plant, but there is no doubt that throughout the Western world, Echinacea is one of the top-selling herbal medicines. Some estimate that the West spent nearly a billion dollars on Echinacea last year.

Welcome to the world of Echinacea. Even those who know little about herbal medicine have heard of Echinacea, and many keep a bottle in the medicine chest. Echinacea has taken the world by storm and people want to know more about it. The book you have in your hands is everything you ever wanted to know about Echinacea, and then some.

Let me introduce myself. I am a qualified medical herbalist specialising in immuno-active medicinal plants, that is plants that improve immune function. Echinacea is one of the many medicinal plants that I am currently studying. It also happens to be one of my favourites.

I have focused my work on the immune system for two reasons. First, I hold it responsible for a host of the health complaints that medical practitioners see today. From AIDS to ME, from rheumatoid arthritis to lupus, the immune system is running amok in the modern age, and causing wide-scale suffering. Second, whereas orthodox medicine offers little to treat diseases based on immune-system failure, the world of herbal medicine is a treasure trove for people who suffer their effects. Plants like Echinacea are a potential solution for millions of people.

I am a part of a think-tank called HCR, which is short for 'The

Herbalists on Columbia Road'. Columbia Road, by the way, is a street in the East End of London. It is home to a very old flower market and to our herbal medicines think-tank. As Great Britain is the only country in the Western world in which the practice of herbal medicine is legal, it has become a Mecca for professionals in the field. In Columbia Road you will also find our clinic and our pharmacy. If you are ever in the area, drop in.

HCR consists of herbalists, doctors, chemists, toxicologists, nurses and other scientific types with an obsession for herbal medicine. We spend our days studying medicinal plants in the lab and in clinical practice. Our objective is to advance the knowledge of herbal medicines as best we can and to pass this knowledge on to the general public. In many ways, this book results from our collective work with Echinacea over the years. It could be called the HCR report on Echinacea. You have in your hands a study put together by experts both in the field of herbal medicine and in science in general.

*   *   *

When I sat down to write I had several objectives in mind. I may as well announce my agenda, since, make no mistake, there is an agenda for this book, and it is fairly clear-cut.

My first objective is to set the record straight. Echinacea is a highly popular herbal medicine and people make all kinds of incredible claims for it. There is a lot of misinformation floating around the subject. Consumers and professionals alike have succumbed to misconceptions, and this bothers me both as a stickler for detail and as a lover of the plant.

Misinformation is always bad. Misinformation about a medicinal plant is dangerous. Echinacea is above all a medicine, and we do not want to be using medicines incorrectly, whether chemical or herbal. My intention is to clarify a situation that has become rather murky, so that people may use this plant correctly. I hope to give the consumer and the practitioner the FACTS.

For better or worse, the herbal medicine industry is unregulated. Consumers are offered no protection by government agencies or self-created regulatory agencies, so with no one looking out for their best interests, they have to protect themselves. Knowing the facts about Echinacea will enable them to do that. My second objective is to give them the information they need to make the right choices.

Here is a classic example. Most indicators we have suggest that the medicinal part of Echinacea is the *root*. Historically speaking, the leaf has never been used as a medicine, and contemporary research suggests that its medicinal value is only marginal. Professionals in the field prefer to use the root. Yet a trip to many health food shops reveals that some of the products sold there are made from Echinacea *leaf*. Why? One non-medical reason might be that the plant yields a whole lot of leaf and not much root. The leaf is cheap, the root is expensive. Whatever the reason, consumers need to be apprised of the facts so that they can make a decision for themselves. This book aims to provide consumers with what is known about Echinacea. If they decide to buy leaf-based products, they will be doing so in the knowledge that they are buying something not traditionally used as medicine.

Three big issues
When I think about Echinacea and what the consumer needs to know, three questions come to mind. The first is: 'Which Echinacea should be used as medicine?' There are several species, and one needs to know which is the best source. The second issue is: 'What is an appropriate use for Echinacea?' People are using the plant for all kinds of conditions, many of which are not improved with its use. The last and final issue is: 'How should Echinacea be used?' Many people are using doses so small that they are about as effective as drinking tap water. Echinacea works when used in appropriate doses. If you want to experience its benefits, you need to know some basic facts about it. Before we move on, let's look at these questions a little more closely.

Which Echinacea should be used medicinally?   In the contemporary marketplace the term 'Echinacea' does not refer to a specific plant but rather to a genus or group of plants. There are eight different species of Echinacea native to North America, a list which includes *Echinacea angustifolia, E. atrorubens, E. laevigata, E. pallida, E. paradoxa, E. purpurea, E. simulata,* and *E. tennesseensis.* Each of these species occupies a different part of the United States and is a different plant.

When you purchase 'Echinacea' at the health food shop or herb store today, you are usually buying a product made from either *E. pallida, E. purpurea* or *E. angustifolia.* These are the most commonly grown species. Some Echinacea products do not indicate which species has been used to make them, so for preference you should choose one that does. Though these related plants are sold as being interchangeable, in fact they are not. When the different Echinacea species were screened chemically, each one turned out to contain a very different cocktail of compounds. If their composition was the same, one could accept the different species being sold as interchangeable. But they are not the same, and should be seen as separate entities. You the consumer should ask: Which species of Echinacea was used to make this product? If the label does not answer your question, move on.

So the big question becomes, which Echinacea species should be used as a medicine? In order to answer the question, my plan is to present the facts regarding the different species and to allow you, the reader, to make your own informed decision. From here on, the different Echinacea species will be identified by their names. Just to refer to 'Echinacea' will not do. These are different plants, and they must be dealt with as such.

What conditions should be treated with the Echinacea species? As I sit in my pharmacy and clinic in London I have a steady stream of people coming through the door looking for this or that herbal medicine. As Echinacea is one of the most popular, thousands of people request it. I always ask them why they need Echinacea before I hand them a bag of the root or a bottle of its tincture, and I am frequently horrified to discover what condition they plan to treat. Too often, their intentions turn out to be downright misguided.

I would estimate that over half of the visitors to my pharmacy intend to use Echinacea for a condition that will absolutely not be improved with its use. Some well-meaning neighbour, aunt or schoolmate tells them that Echinacea will help them with their gall bladder troubles, and without any further investigation, they go out to get some. When they come into my shop they are soon set straight and directed to a more appropriate herbal medicine. Unfortunately, a lot of shops do not question these misguided consumers. Many people are using the wrong medicine for the wrong ailment, and we need to correct this situation.

Thus, to ascertain appropriate use for Echinacea is an important aim of this book. We shall examine the uses of this medicinal plant from its earliest history to the present day. Echinacea is not good for everything. No medicinal plant is. It is good for some conditions and ineffective for others. The point is to learn which is which.

How should the Echinacea species be used as medicine? When you go to a health food shop you will find some 'Echinacea' products made out of the root, some out of the leaf, and sometimes even the stem is used. Some products come as tablets and others in liquid form. Some tell you to take 250 mg a day, others recommend 1000 mg a day. We shall deal with the questions: 'How much?' 'How often?' and 'In what form?'

These three big questions have to be addressed and answered before you head for the health food shop with shopping on your mind. If that means absorbing information, I can promise that the task is worthwhile. I spend my days working with boatloads of medicinal plants and I know a star when I see one. Understanding Echinacea provides us with a powerful medicinal tool. Medicines only work when used correctly. Use diarrhoea medication for a headache, and your headache is not going to go away. If you want to take advantage of this miracle plant (and it is a miracle plant), you have to do a little homework.

On a rather more positive note, having worked with many medicinal plants that stimulate the immune system, I have seen Echinacea do things that no other medicine does. It offers a unique healing option, and one that deserves to be better-known to consumers and health care professionals alike.

General practitioners and patients the world over have been warned that they are no longer to indiscriminately prescribe or use antibiotics. Health agencies around the globe have put out the word that antibiotics are to be reserved for emergency situations only. It is my opinion that Echinacea can be used as a non-antibiotic solution to infection. Hopefully this book will give everyone the information they need to take advantage of this valuable alternative.

The medical profession is clamping down on antibiotic use because fifty years of antibiotic over-prescription have bred a new generation of antibiotic-resistant bacteria. The words 'antibiotic-resistant strain' strike terror down the spines of many health care professionals. People turn up at hospitals with infections that simply do not yield to antibiotics, others leave hospital with infections that no antibiotic can conquer, and their doctors do not know what to do. From the research I have done, it is clear to me that Echinacea offers a logical option and a powerful healing tool to health care practitioners confronting lethal bacteria that will not yield to orthodox treatment.

Antibiotic-resistant strains of bacteria are largely a problem for the West, which has been investing in antibiotics for the last fifty years. In many other parts of the world, people die from bacterial infection simply because they cannot afford antibiotics. For them, Echinacea represents an affordable option. It can be grown readily in many climates, and it acts both to prevent and to cure. Yet for the moment it is not getting much use in the developing world, and this is much to be regretted. Echinacea represents a powerful source of medicine today, and for the future. One of my objectives here is to get people thinking about all of its possible applications. This book is intended as a source of guidance and inspiration!

I would like to mention one more important issue. In compiling this book I have conducted a comprehensive survey of the information available. However, I do not rule out the possibility of having missed something out. If you are sitting on information that is not included in this book, by all means send it my way! What I would say is that there is more than enough information here for the consumer to make an educated purchase.

INTRODUCTION

It should be quite clear from this list of objectives that we have some ground to cover! By the time you finish reading this book you will probably know a lot more about Echinacea than when you started. You will have your own opinions on this plant, which will be based on the facts. You will be fully armed with all the information you need to be a skilled consumer.

For those of you who have never read one of my books, you will now be warned. This is going to be an experience. There may be times when you think to yourself: Where on earth is he going with this? Trust me, we are going somewhere. Looking at a medicinal plant is always a journey, and this book travels far. Herbal medicine is multidisciplinary—it opens lots of scientific fields. It involves a bit of botany, chemistry, medicine, history and more. In due course, we shall dip into all the disciplines necessary to meet the ultimate objective of this book—to gain insight into Echinacea, and to use it effectively.

CHAPTER 1

The Botany of the Echinacea Species

When you look at medicinal plants it is best to start at the beginning. As they are plants, the beginning is always botany. Plants come in families, just as people do. Echinacea comes from the family known as Compositae, the daisy family. Most people know it, because its members are common in the garden. The chrysanthemum, the daisy, the sunflower, the dandelion and the thistle are all members. These 'composites', as they are known to botanists, all have a similarly constructed flower—a cup, with petals ringing it. The typical example is the daisy.

The Compositae family is no run-of-the-mill family. It is packed with medicinal members. Here is a short list of those that are currently used for medicine; plants that you might have come across in your travels. They are: arnica, artichoke, blessed thistle, boneset, calendula, chamomile, coltsfoot, dandelion, Echinacea, milk thistle.

As members of human families have common characteristics, so plant families share commonalties. We have seen that all Compositae have a similarly constructed flower. Another family trait is that many can be used as a medicine. Even more specifically, the 'composites' are used for a similar purpose: calendula, chamomile and arnica are all used to speed healing. In fact, all the Compositae are used to speed healing. Here is our list, showing the various healing actions speeded by the plant:

Arnica: muscles
Artichoke: liver

Blessed thistle: infectious disease
Boneset: infectious disease
Calendula: skin
Chamomile: skin and gut
Coltsfoot: lungs
Dandelion: liver
Echinacea: infectious disease
Milk thistle: liver

Beyond speeding healing, the Compositae have been used to prevent people catching infectious diseases. Blessed thistle was used to keep people from picking up bubonic plague, boneset against coming down with influenza, Echinacea against picking up diphtheria, milk thistle to ward off viral hepatitis. Contemporary research has shown that these plants contain compounds which fire up the immune system to renewed activity. The immune cells are responsible both for healing and fighting off infectious disease. The composites are packed with compounds able to stimulate the immune system.

The next time you come across a daisy relation being used to stimulate healing, or prevent infection, you will not be surprised. The entire family has been used for centuries for those purposes, and modern research has confirmed this use!

As you have already read, 'Echinacea' is a generic term for several species of plants unique to North America—that is, they are only found growing wild on that continent. To refresh your memory, the Echinacea species that can be found growing in different parts of North America are: *E. angustifolia, E. atrorubens, E. laevigata, *E. pallida, E. paradoxa, *E. purpurea, E. simulata, E. tennesseensis. The three species marked with asterisks are the ones you are likely to encounter at the health food or herb shop. The other species are of interest only to academics. Unless you spend your time at botanical conventions you are unlikely ever to come across them.

You have already discovered that many composites are used to stimulate the immune system. The Echinacea species are thought to be the most active immune stimulants in the composite family,

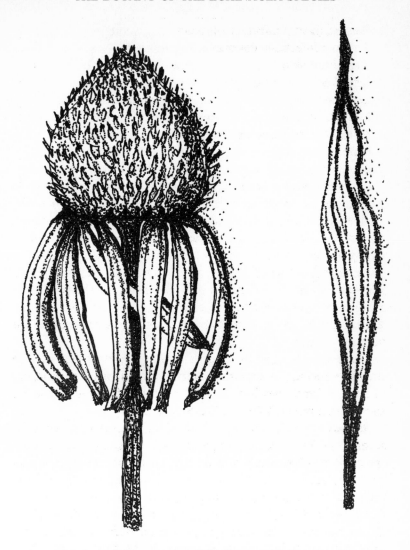

Echinacea angustifolia, flower and leaf.

and the best way to view them is to see them like brothers and sisters with the same parents. Siblings tend to have similar traits. They may have the same eyes or hair colour. Brothers and sisters may be similar, but they will also differ from one another. The same is true for the Echinacea species. In some regards they are

19

similar, in others different—and they are no more interchangeable than a brother and sister are interchangeable.

There are three key points to take away from this discussion of botany. First, various daisy family members have been used for many centuries to speed healing and protect against infectious disease. Second, there are different species of Echinacea and they, like many of their relatives, have been found to improve immune function. Third, while they are naturally similar, the Echinacea species are not identical to one another. They are different plants.

CHAPTER 2

Echinacea and Native American Medicine

One advantage of studying history is that you do not have to spend your time re-inventing the wheel. In most fields of study, a careful review of the past will tell you much of what you need to know. Many of the answers we crave can be found by reviewing the history of the Echinacea species. People have been using the species for hundreds of years, and experience counts. If our objective is to learn which of them should be used as medicine, what conditions that species should be used to treat, and how that plant should be used, we should remember that people in the past have already grappled with these issues.

We at HCR spend a lot of time looking at the historical uses of medicinal plants. Indeed, in order for us to feel good about a herbal medicine, we feel it must have a long history of use. There is a certain comfort to be derived from knowing that a plant has been used for centuries to treat a certain condition. The fact that liquorice has been used for six thousand years to treat respiratory tract infections says something. First, it says that liquorice must improve respiratory function. People would not have used it for so long if it did not work. Second, it tells us that in all those thousands of years, nothing bad has happened to the user. No one has developed harmful symptoms. If liquorice was toxic, people would have noticed years ago. We like plants that have a history.

Likewise, it is a bit worrying for the thinkers at HCR when a plant with no history of use becomes popular and widely used. With plants such as these, we lack long-term assurances. Do they have hidden side-effects? Where plants have not been subjected to the test of time, we are less inclined to have confidence in them. That is not to say that new plants have no merit, but rather that they probably need to undergo the extensive clinical trials that new chemical drugs have to face. The mere fact that they are nature-made does not stamp them as safe.

The chances are that if you are reading this book you are interested in herbal medicine. Some people pick up a romantic novel when they are in a book shop, and you have ended up with a book on Echinacea. If this is the case, looking at the history of a medicinal plant is a skill you need to acquire. Our society stopped using medicinal plants two generations ago. Most of us interested in their revival are starting at ground zero. Not only will the next two chapters reveal lost Echinacea secrets, they will teach you how to review a medicinal plant's history. This is a skill you will use time and time again.

* * *

With regard to the Native American uses of the Echinacea species, one point has to be made clear from the outset. The picture that survives is a vague one. Much of the Native American knowledge of the medicinal plants was lost during the colonial period. This applies to the Echinacea species as to all other American plants. The Native Americans themselves were almost wiped out as a consequence of the draconian policies practised by European colonials who spent far more of their time killing the original inhabitants, stealing their land, and infecting them with diseases than on asking them what plants they used for medicine. As a result, we know only a fraction of what the Native Americans knew about the Echinacea species.

Nevertheless, in the later part of the nineteenth century and the beginning of the twentieth there was a handful of people of European ancestry who took an interest in the Native American plants and ways. One such person was Melvin Randolph Gilmore. In a work published in 1919 by this forward-thinking individual, we find a passage which summarises the situation nicely:

During the period which has elapsed since the European occupancy of the continent of North America there has never been a thoroughgoing, comprehensive survey of the flora with respect to the knowledge of it and its uses possessed by the aboriginal population. Until recent years little study has been made of the ethnobotany of any of the tribes or of any phytogeographic region. Individual studies have been made, but the subject has not claimed a proportionate share of interest with other phases of botanical study. The people of the European race in coming into the New World have not really sought to make friends of the native population, or to make adequate use of the plants or the animals indigenous to this continent, but rather to exterminate everything found here and to supplant it with the plants and animals to which they were accustomed at home.

The European colonials were not interested in the Native Americans or their ways. Much like the coyote and the bobcat, the Native Americans were seen as an inconvenience. The colonials did not document their medicines before they set out to exterminate them. Many tribes were wiped out completely, others survived in part. When the Native Americans died, so did the knowledge they had picked up over the centuries. Looking at the Native American use of Echinacea involves picking through the ashes of what was once a bright fire.

This sad reality would be less dire if the Native American healing tradition had been recorded, that is if the Native Americans had written their knowledge down. Unfortunately, it was an oral tradition: knowledge was passed down from one generation to the next by word of mouth. There are no books dating back thousands of years encapsulating the Native American knowledge once held. When the healers were killed, their knowledge died.

Those Native Americans who were not killed often had Christianity imposed upon them by the incoming European missionaries. This further worsened the situation, because the missionaries actively turned the Native Americans against their own healers and healing ways. The basic reason is a simple one. In Native

American culture the medicine man or woman was also a spiritual practitioner. This made the local healer the enemy of the missionaries, who therefore attempted to undermine their influence on their own people. One way to do this was to devalue their knowledge of the medicinal plants that flourished in their land. The Native Americans were strongly encouraged to reject their own healers and healing ways.

For all these reasons, attempting to trace the Native American use of the Echinacea species prior to the European presence in North America is a challenge. It requires the researcher to piece together bits of information from diverse sources, and all this patchwork effort reminds us how much has been lost along the way. However, some guidance does emerge, and bear in mind that throughout this review we will be looking at information gathered by Europeans. Before we start, I would like to mention an interesting fact. Many manufacturers and professionals are under the impression today that Echinacea was the top medicinal plant of the Native Americans. There is a common belief that it was a cure-all. Research tells a very different story.

EARLY RECORDS

In the early colonial historical record, *Echinacea angustifolia* and *Echinacea purpurea* are the only two species that appear. *E. purpurea* is found growing on the East Coast of the United States, and *E. angustifolia* appears to the West. Not surprisingly, the colonials came across *E. purpurea* first, and it was the first Echinacea to be mentioned in their botanical accounts.

The earliest reference to the Echinacea species is in a book entitled *Flora Virginica*, published in 1762 by L. T. Gronovius and based on the field observations of an English botanist by the name of John Clayton, who lived from 1693 to 1773. Clayton lived in Virginia for forty years, and there he came across *Echinacea purpurea*. In his notes we see that *E. purpurea* was used to treat saddle sores on horses. Whether or not this was a Native American practice is unknown. The chances are that the suggestion came from the soon-to-be-exterminated Native Americans living in Virginia.

In the early colonial days, European botanists did spend time travelling around taking notes about the plants they came across. They were plant adventurers if you will. One of the most important was a man named Raffinesque, whose custom was to pay special attention to the plants widely used by the Native Americans as medicine, and to the purposes for which they would be used. In 1830, Raffinesque mentions that the Sioux Indians used *E. angustifolia* to treat syphilis. That is all he has to say about it, and the very fact that he had so little to say about this medicinal plant seriously challenges the notion that the 'Echinacea species' was the Native American cure-all and preferred medicinal plant. Had it been widely used, Raffinesque would have taken note, as he did about a lot of other plants.

In 1835 a much-quoted authority named Riddell remarked of *E. purpurea*: 'root thick, black, very pungent to the taste, aromatic, carminative, little known'. In 1848 the botanist Asa Gray mentions *E. purpurea* in his *Manual of Botany* and remarks that it is known in domestic medicine as black sampson and it is used by quack doctors. Once again, this record does not tell us a lot about the Native American use of the species.

Our next titbit comes from a rather interesting source—the Shakers. They were an unconventional religious cult who are usually associated with furniture-making, though in fact this was a sideline in their way of life. The original Shakers left England to found health farms in the New World. They felt that life in London was bad for the health, and looked to the American frontier as a refuge from the smog and filth of London. Once arrived on the other side, they set up the health farms conceived in the squalor of the London slums.

In Shaker communes, marriage was discouraged and procreation frowned upon. The founder felt there was nothing natural about copulation. People spent their days collecting medicinal plants and manufacturing medicines. Unlike most of the European colonists, they actively pursued the Native Americans to learn what plants could be used for medicine. Amongst other things, the Shakers kept extremely accurate records, and these give us clues as to how the Native Americans used the Echinacea species, and indeed many other medicinal plants.

To begin with, the Shakers used *E. angustifolia*, which they began to collect and brew into medicine in 1837. They viewed it as a useful medicine in urinary complaints—information that would have come straight to them via the Native Americans. Sadly, the Shakers did not have more to say. Once again, we have a challenge to the notion that Echinacea was the favourite Native American plant.

LATER HISTORY

At the turn of the twentieth century a group of individuals realised that the Native American culture was in danger. So they banded together and lobbied Congress to set up an agency to record Native American knowledge before it disappeared outright. In response, the American Congress established the Bureau of American Ethnology, whose mission was to catalogue the knowledge of the Native Americans before their culture entirely vanished. Field researchers travelled to the remnants of what were once great tribes and collected information from them. Much of what we know about the Native American use of Echinacea comes from the efforts of the ethnographers working for this department.

Melvin Randolf Gilmore was one of the individuals who went out and learned from the Native Americans. In a paper he published in 1913, 'A Study in the Ethnobotany of the Omaha Indians', we find reference to one of the Echinacea species being used as medicine. Gilmore refers to:

> ... *Echinacea angustifolia*, the uses of which the Indians of the plains have known for ages ... Of plants used medicinally, one of the greatest importance is *Echinacea angustifolia*, called I'n'Shtogahtehi in reference to its use for sore eyes; called also mika ega'n'tashi, in reference to the use of its spiny cone for a comb by children in play. In medicine the part used was the root, macerated and applied as an antidote for snake bites, stings, and all septic diseases. It was applied to the hands and arms by the 'mystery men' as a local anaesthetic to deaden sensation so that they might

26

remove pieces of meat from the boiling pot without flinching, thus manifesting their supernatural power and so obtaining influence over the credulous. Two kinds were distinguished as Nuga, male, and Miga, female; the apparent differences being the size, Nuga being larger, and the small size or Miga being considered the efficient medicine. A common ailment among the Omaha is eye trouble, and for all its alleviation various agents were employed, among them being the root of *Echinacea angustifolia*, the hips of *Rosa arkansana*, and various other plants.

This text is revealing in several regards. We learn from it that the Omaha tribe used *E. angustifolia* to treat poisonous bites, infected wounds, and infected eyes. This use of the plant to treat wounds and infection is one that will reappear time and time again. We also see that it was used to deaden the pain of burns, a use that has been entirely forgotten in the modern age (though it does work!).

The same writer refers to Echinacea in a later text, 'Uses of Plants by the Indians of the Missouri River Region', published in 1918. By this time he has learned more about *E. angustifolia*. He tells us that the plant was known to the Dakota tribe as Ichalipe-hu or whip plant. The Omaha-Ponca tribe called it Mika-hi, which means comb plant. The same tribe called the plant isthagalite-hi when it was being used to treat eye conditions. The Pawnee called it Ksapitahako, meaning whirling hands plant. Here we have three more tribes using *E. angustifolia* for medicine, each with a different name for the plant.

The rest of Gilmore's report is worth quoting at length:

This plant was universally used as an antidote for snake bite and other venomous bites and stings and poisonous conditions. Echinacea seems to have been used as a remedy for more ailments than any other plant. It was employed in the smoke treatment for headache in persons and distemper in horses It was used also as a remedy for toothache, a piece being kept on the painful tooth until there was relief, and for

27

enlarged glands, as in mumps. It was said that jugglers bathed their hands and arms in the juice of this plant so that they could take out a piece of meat from a boiling kettle with the bare hand without suffering pain, to the wonderment of onlookers. A Winnebago said that he often used the plant to make his mouth insensible to heat, so that for show he could take a live coal in his mouth. Burns were bathed with the juice to give relief from the pain, and the plant was used in the steam bath to render the great heat endurable.

The tragedy of this text is that the author tells us that *Echinacea angustifolia* was used by these tribes for more conditions than any other plant, and then does not document their use! Incidentally, Gilmore is the only historian to report that *Echinacea angustifolia* was widely used by the Native Americans.

Our next reference to the Echinacea species comes from an article entitled, 'Ethnobotany of the Meskwaki Indians'. It was written by Huron Smith in 1928 and appeared in a publication from the Public Museum of the City of Milwaukee. Once again *E. angustifolia* is the species used as medicine. Concerning the medicinal practices of these two tribes, we read that: 'The root is used in medicine to cure cramps in the stomach and also to cure fits. The freshly scraped root was used by the Sioux Indians as a remedy for hydrophobia, snakebite, and septic conditions.' The author tells us that the Prairie Potowatami specifically used the plant to treat the chronic skin condition known as eczema.

In yet another text, 'Uses of Plants by the Chippewa Indians', written by Frances Densmore in 1928 for the Bureau of American Ethnology, we find that the Chippewa tribe used *E. angustifolia* to treat diseases of horses, burns, and indigestion. The Chippewa tribe lived around the Great Lakes.

Up to this point, we have learned about the Echinacea species through mentions in old texts. We can also draw conclusions from texts where it is *not* mentioned. There is a text called the Swimmer Manuscript, another document published by the Bureau of American Ethnology, a comprehensive survey of the Cherokee tribes' healing practices. It goes on for hundreds of pages in the most elaborate detail. The Cherokees would have had access to *E. purpurea* in the southern United States, and yet there is not a single reference in the Swimmer Manuscript to its use as a medicine. There are lots of drugs listed for the treatment of snakebite; *E. purpurea* is not one of them. This lack of mention suggests that *E. purpurea* may not have been considered all that medicinal by the Native Americans living on the East Coast.

I am afraid to say that we have now exhausted the available hard evidence about Native American use of the Echinacea species. Whether or not the species was a major Native American medicine is unknown. A more accurate statement would be that we know the Native Americans used Echinacea to a limited extent. Now is the time to get back to our initial questions.

WHICH ECHINACEA SPECIES DID THE NATIVE AMERICANS USE AS MEDICINE?

Records of the Native American use of the Echinacea species give pride of place to *Echinacea angustifolia*. From the minimal information available, we know for sure that the Native Americans used the plant as a medicine. Several historians confirm this fact.

On the other hand, there are no records that the Native Americans used *E. purpurea* or *E. pallida*. When the colonials came across *E. purpurea* on the East Coast, they did not record its use as a medicine by the indigenous people. For instance, the Cherokees lived along the East Coast, and yet the Swimmer Manuscript, the authority on Cherokee medicine, makes no mention of *E. purpurea*. This strongly suggests they did not use it.

It follows that if you want advice from the Native Americans, the only concrete recommendation is for *Echinacea angustifolia*. Many people assert that the Echinacea species were all used by the Native Americans as medicine. The hard evidence suggests otherwise. The few records mentioning Echinacea and the Native Americans in the same breath refer to *E. angustifolia*. The tribes not surveyed in detail may have used the other species: we shall never know. We only have factual evidence for *E. angustifolia*.

WHAT CONDITIONS DID THE NATIVE AMERICANS TREAT WITH *ECHINACEA ANGUSTIFOLIA*?

The Native American uses of *E. angustifolia* fall into three major groups or categories. It was seen as an agent that stimulated healing, a painkiller, and a treatment for two infectious diseases. Here are the specific conditions treated with *E. angustifolia*:

Healing agent	*Painkiller*	*Treatment for*
sore eyes	deaden the pain of	*infectious disease*
diseases of the eye	burns	enlarged glands
snakebite	reduce sensations of	mumps
stings	heat	rabies
infected wounds/	headache	
septic disease	toothache	
eczema	stomach ache	
burns	cramps	
	indigestion	
	epilepsy	

From our earlier discussion of the Daisy family, the uses as a healing agent and as a treatment in infectious disease come as no great surprise. They fall in line with the rest of the family. The use on the nervous system is very interesting, and is also a family trait. A cup of soothing chamomile is one of the most famous calming agents in the West. The colonials did come across the uses of *E. angustifolia* in healing and to counter infectious disease. They did not pick up on its use as a painkiller.

HOW DID THE NATIVE AMERICANS USE *ECHINACEA ANGUSTIFOLIA*?

The texts available tell us two things about the Native American use of *E. angustifolia* as a medicine. The first is that they used the root. The second is that they used it fresh. Though the Native Americans did gather some medical substances and dry them for later use, *E. angustifolia* was not one of them. This plant was dug up and the root applied fresh. Specifically, the fresh root was chewed up and either the mush applied or the resulting juice swallowed. We have no records telling us how many roots were to be used or how often. Again, we can only lament the damage inflicted on an entire system of medical practice.

CHAPTER 3

Echinacea angustifolia and the Eclectic School of Medicine

Though Echinacea had probably been in use for thousands of years before the Eclectic School of Medicine started working with it, the Eclectics were responsible for introducing it to the official medical world, and to the world in general. These odd-ball physicians worked diligently with the Echinacea species, so their practice and thoughts are very relevant to those interested in using this group of plants today. Learning about Echinacea means delving into the world of the Eclectic physicians, and body of knowledge they left behind. To this day, they are our principal source of clinical information.

The Eclectic medical movement started on the East Coast of the United States in 1845, in protest against the practices of the medical establishment of the day. Its founder and leader was Wooster Beach. When Dr Beach first started his medical practice, leeches, bleeding, purging, cautery, and heavy metals such as mercury and lead were in vogue amongst medical practitioners as 'healing tools'. Sick patients were routinely bled, burnt and poisoned, to within an inch of their life, supposedly to cure them. Wooster Beach took issue with these practices, which to his mind were sick, perverted, and contrary to key laws of nature.

Wooster Beach believed that the physician should work in tune with the body and with nature to stimulate healing, rather than against the grain. He felt that any medicine or medical procedure that diminished the vital force or strength of the organism was better avoided. Instead, he preferred to use plants, because they were mild and did not damage the body. True to his convictions, he set up a medical school that preached working with nature, rather than against it.

Wooster Beach was practising medicine in New York City in the 1840s, and that is where he set up his school of natural medicine. None too pleased with this group of radical physicians who dared to question the medical authority of the day, the medical establishment went out of its way to make life a misery for Beach and his colleagues. Early on, he and his fellow reformers were taunted, abused and ridiculed. At the time, all they were saying was that bleeding people to the point of death was contrary to nature. However, then, as now, when you contradict medical establishments, storms must follow.

Eventually the medical reformers lost patience with their persecutors and decided to move their school to the remote regions of the West, where there was no medical establishment to bother them. At that time the new Ohio territory was being colonised, and land was on offer to those who would come and take it. Wooster Beach secured a place in Ohio where he and his friends could practise the medicine they believed in, unmolested. Worthington, Ohio, was the first home of the medical reformers, and it was there that the term 'Eclectic' was first applied to their medicine. In time, their new Eclectic Institute would become a great medical centre.

Now it happens that Ohio is home to all three most commonly mentioned species of Echinacea, and it was there that the Eclectics first came into contact with the plant. As we have seen, the Echinacea species had been used by the Native Americans, for a variety of ailments, for centuries. When the Eclectics landed in the Midwest, they met people who told them that these plants could be used in cases of infectious disease, inflammations, rattlesnake bites, and slow-healing wounds. These tips did not fall on deaf ears. The Eclectics were trying to forge a new medical practice and they were looking for new medicines.

Although at first the Eclectics used *E. angustifolia* for the same purposes as the Native Americans did, over time they applied it to an ever-growing list of conditions, with varying success. One special distinction of their movement is that they kept records, wrote books, and carefully documented the knowledge they gained. In our quest for the uses of the Echinacea species, we shall look at their textbooks from the beginning of the movement to the end. The Eclectics were the masters of Echinacea. They worked with it longer and harder than any other group of people in the history of the world. Studying their books is the best way to get to know this plant. We shall review some key texts.

*　　*　　*

Wooster Beach, *The Medical and Botanical Dictionary*, published by the author, New York 1847
At the time this book was published, Echinacea was known as Rudbeckia, and it is under that name we find it listed. Dr Beach lists four varieties of Rudbeckia, *R. fulgida*, *R. lanciniata*, *R. purpurea*, and *R. triloba*. One of the problems with studying herbal medicines, is that botanists have an infuriating habit of changing plant names. The Echinacea species fall into this category. In 1847 the Eclectics had not long been in the Midwest, and Beach's complete silence as to their medicinal attributes tells us that they had not learned of their medicinal virtues. This makes sense. The Eclectics reached Ohio after most of the Native Americans of that region had been killed, or moved on. There was plenty of Echinacea growing there. Unfortunately, those who knew how to use it were gone.

*　　*　　*

John King, MD, *The American Eclectic Dispensatory*, Moore, Wilstach, and Keys, Cincinnati 1854
In one of the first comprehensive texts of Eclectic medicines, 'King's Dispensatory', we see the first medicinal use of Echinacea listed. The text that would become the Bible of the Eclectics records their use of *E. angustifolia* for kidney disorders, and *E.*

purpura for syphilis. It is a fairly short list of uses. At the time Echinacea was clearly a minor player in the Eclectic repertoire of medicines. What matters is that they initially used both species as medicine. The references are as follows:

Echinacea angustifolia. This plant grows in various parts of the United States, in damp places, low thickets, edges of swamps, ditches, etc., flowering from July to September. The whole herb is recommended to be used. Its chemical reactions, as well as formation, are not known. It imparts its properties to water.

Thimbleweed [Echinacea] is a valuable diuretic, tonic, and balsamic. Useful in many diseases of the urinary organs, and highly recommended in strangury, Bright's disease, and wasting and atrophy of the kidneys. Dose of the decoction, ad libitum.

Echinacea purpurea. The *Rudbeckia purpurea* of Linnaeus, variously called red sunflower, comb flower, or purple coneflower (the *Echinacea purpurea* of Moenchhausen), has a thick, black root. This plant is common to the western prairies and banks, and is found also in the Southern States flowering from July to September. The root is very pungent to the taste, and has been popularly used in medicine under the name black sampson; it is stated to have been employed with much benefit in syphilis.

Though the Eclectics' use of Echinacea was still minimal, we can see an increase in their knowledge. To summarise King's account of these two plants, he mentions their use in diseases of the urinary organs, lack of urine production, kidney disease, wasting and atrophy of the kidneys, chronic bacterial infection, and syphilis. He also makes a very interesting recommendation at the end of his discussion: 'Both of the above plants, deserve a full and thorough investigation from the profession. From all I have been able to learn, the latter plant is equal to stillingia in medicinal efficacy.' Clearly the good doctor had noticed there was something special about these plants.

However, this is one of the first and last times that we will read about *E. purpurea* being used as a medicine by the group. This species had only a brief season in the sun with the Eclectics. From here on, we shall only read about *E. angustifolia* being used as a medicine.

*   *   *

Wooster Beach, *The American Practice Condensed*, Moore, Wilstach, and Keys, Cincinnati 1869
Here again, Wooster Beach mentions one of the Echinacea species, though very briefly. In this text he talks about *E. angustifolia*, and does not say a word about the other species he wrote about previously. Here is what he has to say:

> Thimbleweed (*Rudbeckia laccinata*)   Diuretic and balsamic; recommended in wasting diseases of the kidneys; given freely, in decoction.

We don't see anything new here, but rather a rehash of Dr King's account. It is curious that these early references talk about *E. angustifolia* being used to treat kidney disease. This is a use you will not find amongst modern herbalists.

*   *   *

As we approach the year 1885, the Echinacea plot thickens.

When the white population started moving Westward in North America, they often found themselves in places that lacked the necessities of life. Minister, doctors, lawmen and teachers were in short supply out West, and self-appointed doctors were commonplace—men who had no medical training apart from having spent some time working with a doctor. When you were suffering from a gunshot wound, or had trouble delivering a child, a self-appointed doctor was better than no doctor at all.

One such 'doctor', Dr Meyer from Pawnee, Nebraska, was largely responsible for widening the Eclectic use of *E. angustifolia*. He may not have been medically trained, and indeed some texts suggest that he was illiterate. All the same we have him to thank for forcing the Eclectics to take it more seriously.

The following lines are excerpted from an Eclectic medical book written by a Dr Felter. He tells the tale of how this 'country doctor' put *E. angustifolia* in the mind of every Eclectic.

The introduction of Echinacea into professional practice is due conjointly to Dr. H. F. C. Meyer, of Pawnee City, Neb., and the late Prof. John King. The former had, for many years . . . been using the plant without knowing its botanical position. In a letter to Prof. King . . . in 1886, he communicated to the latter his uses of the drug, as he had employed it for 16 years. His claims for the remedy were based upon the conclusion that it was 'an antispasmodic and antidote for blood-poisoning'.

The enthusiastic doctor had been using it in a secret mixture with wormwood and hops, which he had denominated 'Meyer's Blood Purifier'. Among his claims for it, was its antidotal action upon the poison of various insects, and particularly that of the rattlesnake. Meyer stated that he even allowed a rattler to bite him, after which he bathed the parts with some of the tincture, took a drachm of it internally, and laid down and slept, and upon awakening all traces of swelling had disappeared! . . .

The following range of affections were those in which Dr Meyer claimed success for this remedy: Malarial fever, cholera morbus, cholera infantum, boils, and internal abscesses, typhoid fever (internally and locally to abdomen); ulcerated sore throat, old ulcers, poisoning from rhus, erysipelas, carbuncles, bites and stings of bees, wasps, spiders, etc.; in nasal and pharyngeal catarrh, haemorrhoids, various fevers, including typhoid, congestive, and remittent; trichinosis, nervous headache, acne, scrofulous ophthalmia, milk crust, scald head, and eczema; also in colic in horses.

Subsequent use of the drug has in a measure substantiated the seemingly incredulous claims of its introducer, for it will be observed that most of the conditions were such as might be due to blood depravation, or to noxious introductions from without the body—the very field in which Echinacea is known to display its power.

Fortunately, the Eclectics listened to the message, overlooked their scepticism about the messenger, and took the information on board. As we have seen, Dr King, one of the movers and shakers within the movement, had earlier expressed his interest in Echinacea. He had been waiting to learn more, and Dr Meyer gave him the opportunity.

Before we look at what Dr Meyer said about *E. angustifolia*, we should ask where he got the information. You may have noted that he lived in Pawnee, Nebraska. Pawnee is the name of a tribe of Native Americans. He worked and lived amongst a large Native American population, and he recommended its being used the way the Native Americans used it. In other words, what Dr Meyer really did was to provide the Eclectics with the Native Americans' knowledge of this plant.

Dr Meyer passed on two precious bits of information to the Eclectics. The first was that Echinacea was an effective treatment in infectious disease and venomous bites. The second was that it was *E. angustifolia* that should be used in medical practice. In fact Dr Meyer did not know which Echinacea he was using, but Dr King was a stickler for detail. He had the drug used by Meyer analysed and identified the plant in question. *Echinacea angustifolia* would be the Eclectic choice when it came to the Echinacea species.

*　　*　　*

I. J. M. Goss, MD, *The Practice of Medicine on the Specific Art of Healing*, W. T. Keener, Chicago 1888
Shortly after Dr Meyer's contact with the Eclectics, we find positive proof that they took him seriously. In Dr Goss's book we find that *E. angustifolia* is now being recommended to treat two

infectious diseases: rabies and syphilis. Beyond this, he recommends it being used to treat snakebite. No mystery as to whence this enlightenment came. Here is what Goss had to say:

Snake bite: 'Recently I have been informed by Dr Meyer, of Pawnee City, Nebraska that the *Echinacea angustifolia* is a positive remedy.'

Ulcers: 'It is a fine stimulant, and at the same time it has proved a fine antiseptic in indolent ulcers, etc.'

Syphilis: 'I use Echinacea with iodide of potassium, dose a teaspoonful three times a day. Recently I have been testing *Echinacea angustifolia* and have found it a most potent remedy. I make saturated tincture of the fresh root, crushed, and give thirty to 60 drops three times a day. This has proved with me, one of the most active antisyphilitics, and will give satisfactory results.'

Rabies: 'I have recently treated two cases that were bitten by a rabid dog in this city, with *Echinacea angustifolia*, and neither of them have had any signs of hydrophobia; but the same dog bit another dog, which was not treated, and the bitten dog became rabid in due time, and was killed, I learned. This is doubtless a very valuable remedy in this disease, and as a preventative.'

In this text we have evidence that the Eclectics took Meyer seriously and that they applied what he knew. But they did more than just follow the information they were handed. They explored and refined it. We see this in this first text following Meyer's contact with the Eclectics.

For the most part, Goss simply echoes Dr Meyer's reports. However, he also presents us with important information about the use of *E. angustifolia*, based on his experience with it. He tells us that a saturated tincture should be made of the fresh root. (Saturated tinctures were a minimum of a 1.1 ratio, if not stronger—that is, they were made of one part Echinacea root and one part alcohol.) Goss also says that it should be prescribed in large amounts: 3 millilitres of this saturated tincture three times a day. His message was, use *E. angustifolia* strong and frequently. When we are trying to resurrect herbal medicine, it is important to resurrect it accurately. This doctor's recommendation of using strong and often should be taken on board.

*   *   *

J. S. Neiderkorn, MD , *The Physician's and Student's Ready Guide to Specific Medication*, The Little Printing Company, Bradford, Ohio 1892
Medicinal applications listed in the text:

Acute bacterial infection: diphtheria, typhoid, cholera infantum, septicaemia.

Chronic bacterial infections: tuberculosis, syphilis.

Healing: old wounds, sores.

Neiderkorn describes *Echinacea angustifolia* as: 'An alterative of great value in strumous diathesis, syphilis, old sores and wounds, a powerful antiseptic, locally and internally, in diphtheria, typhoid conditions, cholera infantum, and in blood poisoning.'

Here we find that the Eclectics have been experimenting with *E. angustifolia*. Previously, it had been used to treat syphilis, a chronic bacterial infection. Now we see it being used to treat another chronic bacterial infection, tuberculosis, as well as a hand-ful of acute bacterial infections. Both represent a big leap in use for *E. angustifolia* and show that the Eclectics were learning more about this plant through trial and error.

Necessity is the mother of invention, and necessity caused this widened use of *E. angustifolia*. When the Eclectics first landed in Ohio, there were not many people living there. The Native Americans had been either wiped out, or driven out. Towns were just setting up and were sparsely populated. This desolate period did not last long. Wave after wave of immigrants filled these towns. Population swelled, and with this increased number of human beings came an increase in infectious disease. Sewers did not exist, and the contents of bedpans were routinely thrown out of the window!

In the 1890s, the Ohio towns were ravaged by diphtheria, cholera, typhoid, and streptococcal infections. The Eclectics were suddenly confronted with infectious disease, and had to find something to counter it. They had used *E. angustifolia* to treat syphilis for over forty years and had found it effective, so they tried it in cases of epidemic bacterial infections such as cholera and typhoid, and found that it worked. They began describing *E. angustifolia* as an antiseptic, a substance that cleared up bacterial infection.

In Neiderkorn's text, we see gangrene and septicaemia, that is bacterial infection in the blood, being treated with *E. angustifolia*. Life on the range was an active affair, driving fence posts and rounding up cattle. People cut themselves, and in the insanitary environment, infections developed. Often a wound would lead to gangrene. Even more sinister, the bacteria would spread from a wound to the blood. Before this new treatment was used, such scenarios resulted in amputation or death. By 1892 the Eclectics had discovered that all of the above could be avoided when *E. angustifolia* was applied topically and used internally. The plant provided an effective treatment for all types of bacterial infection.

In Dr Neiderkorn's manual we see *E. angustifolia* described as an alterative for the first time. This is very important, as it tells us that the Eclectics had found another use for the plant. To explain what the term 'alterative' meant to the Eclectics, generally speaking, alteratives were defined as drugs that altered the usual course of a disease. When they were used, what you would expect to happen, did not happen.

Here are two examples of how alteratives were used. Syphilis and tuberculosis were chronic bacterial infections that, when left untreated, usually ended in a slow and painful death. Gradually, the patient's health deteriorated until life was snuffed out. The Eclectics noticed that when *E. angustifolia* was used, patients got better and stayed well. *E. angustifolia* altered the usual outcome of these bacterial diseases.

*   *   *

41

Lyman Watkins, MD, *An Eclectic Compendium of the Practice of Medicine*, John M. Scudder's Sons, Cincinnati 1895

The Eclectics were keen on something known as specific medication, and this concept permeates their work. They felt that a doctor should know his drugs inside and out, and be able to assess both when a medicine was indicated or called for, and when it was contra-indicated. It seems a common-sense notion, but at the time many doctors did not really know their drugs and used them rather indiscriminately. The Eclectics sought to pinpoint the uses of a medicinal plant, and in their books you will find 'specific indication' listed frequently. It meant that they had studied the plant closely, and were clear on its powers.

In Dr Watkins's text, we find the specific indication for *E. angustifolia*. Here we see the cases in which the Eclectics felt that the plant was specifically required. This important piece of writing shows us the light in which the Eclectics saw *E. angustifolia* at the turn of the century:

> Strumous (tb) and syphilitic diathesis, ulceration with profuse secretion, tendency to systemic poisoning, foul phagedenic ulcers, diarrhoea with nausea and vomiting, profuse and bad smelling discharges, purplish skin with bluish shining appearance, vesicular eruptions, viscid exudations, painful superficial irritations, burning of surface, breath offensive, dusky coloured mucous membranes, profuse acrid saliva, tendency to gangrene and sloughing, weakness and emaciation.

The person thus described is in serious trouble. For a patient fitting this description, Doctor Watkins advises *E. angustifolia*. We are not talking about someone with a cough or a cold, someone experiencing a dip in health; this man or woman is losing the battle with the elements.

Now is the time to introduce an important concept. If you place a piece of meat on the back patio and leave it there, after a few weeks it is gone. 'Nature', in the form of flies, bacteria, fungi and the like, quickly transforms the Sunday roast into just about nothing. The natural world is filled with organisms which decompose life forms back into soil. Harsh as it may seem, every day the forces of nature that reduce our Sunday roast to a pile of mulch are acting on each and every one of us. When we are in a stage of good health, our life force, vibrancy or vitality beats nature. However, when our health or vitality diminishes, disease starts creeping in. In this 'specific indication' left to us by Dr Watkins, we see that the Eclectics felt that when the body was no longer able to beat the elements, *E. angustifolia* ought be called to the case.

This may seem rather bizarre, but in fact you have probably had experience of this yourself. If you are run down, tired, over-worked and stressed out, your body is not able to fight off disease. Moreover, you may have known someone whose health was failing. In that situation, you no doubt saw the person contract infection after infection. The Eclectics saw the same thing with their patients. When the body was unable to resist, they called upon *E. angustifolia*. They found it stimulated well-being, where it had declined. A health and vitality stimulator has many uses, as you will see as we move along the Eclectic time-line.

*   *   *

H. T. Webster, *Dynamical Therapeutics—A work devoted to the Theory and Practice of Specific Medication with special references to the newer remedies*, 2nd edition 1898
Medicinal applications listed in the text:

Acute bacterial infections: cholera infantum, cholera morbus, diphtheria, dysentery, erysipelas, follicular tonsillitis, perityphilitis, septicaemia, typhoid fever, typhoid fever: septic phase, typhus fever.

Chronic bacterial infections: intermittent, remittent, and chronic fevers; syphilis.

Protozoal infections: malaria, giardia.

Viral infections: measles, smallpox, rabies.

Poisoning: bee sting, poison ivy, rattlesnake bite, venomous snake-bite, miscellaneous causes.

Healing: boils, carbuncles, gangrene, haemorrhoids, pus-filled cavities, ulcerated lower extremities, ulcerated sore throat.

Auto-immune disease: irritable skin conditions.

In this classic text, one of the more noted Eclectics, Dr Webster, lists *E. angustifolia* as one of his favourite medicines, and one that he found to be incredibly dynamic:

> This remedy promises to fill one of the most important pur-poses of any of this class. It is comparatively a new one, but has already afforded eminent satisfaction to quite a large number of Eclectics as a corrector of depraved states of the blood, where ordinary remedies have failed to satisfy the demand.

Dr Webster's book is interesting in that he quotes other Eclectic physicians from around America. His book gives us a window into the ever-widening Eclectic use of *E. angustifolia.*

Previously, we have discussed the uses of *E. angustifolia* in the battle with bacteria. Dr Webster's in-depth case histories—a great way to learn about a medicinal plant—demonstrate its wider appli-cations.

Tarantula bite

> [In 1890] a rancher from San Bernardino county applied to me for relief from effects of a tarantula bite on the hand . . . The bite had been inflicted more than a month before I saw the hand, and plenty of time had elapsed for the effects of the poison to become manifested locally. The middle finger of the right hand over the dorsal aspect of the first phalanx, presented a purplish, sloughing ulcer, as large as a silver quarter, and the whole finger was enormously swollen its entire length, and presented a bluish, shiny appearance. The entire hand was purple and oedematous, while the patient

was worn and emaciated from the constitutional effects of the poison and loss of rest resulting from the local discomfort. The home doctor had treated the case from the beginning, but nothing used had seemed to afford any benefit.

Thus I gave the agent singly, determined to allow it a fair field and no favours. On the second day afterward I saw the hand, and was surprised at the evidence of improvement already visible; and within a week the angry appearance was all gone and ulcer nearly healed. All the malignant aspects of the case had given way, and a few days more sufficed to send the patient on his way rejoicing.

Blood poisoning

I was called to a case with a history of blood poisoning . . . a man sixty-five years of age. Two physicians had given him up. I was much inclined to follow their example, but thought it a good case to test *Echinacea angustifolia* . . . Examination revealed a mass of dead flesh between the metacarpal bones of the index finger and thumb of the right hand. Lifting it, the metacarpal bone lay bare the whole length, both extensor and flexor muscles having sloughed off. The old man was very weak and exhibited the characteristic symptoms of severe poisoning, so I dismissed the thought of amputation and applied the *Echinacea angustifolia* locally, diluting it one-half; also gave it internally full strength. At the end of a week the patient was out of bed.

The other day he walked into my office and exhibited his hand. The chasm was pretty well filled with healthy flesh, the bone being visible at only one small point, the edges of the wound contracted, and so covered with skin that it is reduced to less than one-third its former dimensions. Several times during the treatment I withdrew the internal medicine. Every attempt was followed in a short time by sloughing at some point.

Dr Webster found that even severely infected wounds packed with *E. angustifolia* could recover. He also describes three cases of clear-cut gangrene being cleared with its use. To stress the relevance of these case histories, one has to remember that in those days antibiotics did not exist. Gangrenous wounds meant amputation or death.

When one reviews the reality of the West—poisonous snakes, spiders, scorpions, infectious disease—one realises how desperate many of those that went West must have been. One of the best examples of the horror of the frontier was poison ivy. It is an attractive-looking plant, with lush green leaves and a bushy habit, but its looks are very deceptive. One brush against the plant and your skin melts, literally. The skin becomes red, inflamed, and unbearably painful. In a few short days blisters develop and start to ooze. This is followed by open wounds that take weeks to heal. In the case histories of Dr Webster we find reference to *E. angustifolia* being used to treat the poisoning of this dread plant, 'rhus poisoning' as it was known in those days. Here is one such account:

> I have recently been using *Echinacea angustifolia* in an aggravated case of rhus poisoning, which in California sometimes results in serious consequences. A year before, the patient, a youth who had been in the habit of going into the mountains with dogs and chasing rabbits . . . while breaking through the chaparral thickly lined with the shrub, was confined to his bed for three weeks suffering excruciatingly with the burning and itching all over the body, while his face was swollen beyond recognition. The following season he repeated the rabbit hunt and was again severely poisoned but was only confined to bed for a week. Echinacea was used internally, and as a bath, several times a day upon this occasion, the alcohol vapour bath being employed in connection with it. Since that time he has been exposed to the same influence with complete immunity from the poisonous effects of the scrub, several times.

This case history reminds us that one of the earliest uses of *E. angustifolia* was to counter poisoning in general. When a rattlesnake, scorpion, or poison ivy plant injects its venom into the body, the venom kills the tissue it touches. The result is a black patch or dead tissue around the point of contact with the venom. This might not be such a big deal if the gangrenous patch was on the finger, but if it was, say, in the middle of the stomach, the problem is obvious. The Eclectics noticed that in all of these poisonous bites or brushes, when *E. angustifolia* was used, gangrene did not set in. They did not understand how it did this, but, they did not care. It worked and they used it.

Diphtheria

One of the primary uses of *E. angustifolia* by the Eclectics was against diphtheria. Diphtheria is caused by the bacterium *Cornebacterium diphtheriae* and usually presents at first as a case of tonsillitis, but soon the case worsens, when the bacteria begin to produce toxic compounds that damage cells in the body. These toxic substances first attack the nervous system and ultimately all the other cells in the body, with deadly effects. Dr Webster gives several case histories, some his own and others borrowed, establishing *E. angustifolia*'s effect in diphtheria infection.

Dr. Hayes, of Denver, Colorado, reported six cases of malignant diphtheria cured by this agent . . . The first one he considered hopeless, and so informed the parents; but to his surprise, the patient, a girl twelve years of age, recovered upon being administered *Echinacea angustifolia*, being convalescent in four days. The auxiliary treatment consisted of the inhalation of oil of eucalyptus, evaporated in hot water.

I have used it in one seemingly hopeless case of diphtheria with complete success. In another, where the evidence of malignant blood poisoning was pronounced by marked exhaustion, extensive exudation and sloughing of the fauces, the patient was tided through to convalescence upon *Echinacea angustifolia*, but was afterward killed by injudicious feeding. Another genuine case—and this means a severe one—

recovered promptly upon *Echinacea angustifolia*, and still another which had been saturated with the drug for several days previous to the onset, perished from blocking of the respiratory passages with exudate. . . . These four are the only genuine cases met with between the reading of the report referred to and this writing, but I have formed a very favourable opinion of the remedy from this limited experience.

By this time, the Eclectics knew that the diphtheria bug killed because it produced 'venom' or toxins which caused the illness at hand. As *E. angustifolia* had been so effective in other forms of poisoning, it may explain why they called upon it to treat diphtheria.

Dr Webster also recommended *E. angustifolia* in cases of typhoid fever, which is an infectious disease spread by house lice, and a common killer on the Western frontier. The bacteria produced extremely high body temperatures which caused brain damage in the young, that is if they survived. The Eclectics found that the temperature came down when *E. angustifolia* was employed. They also used the plant against various infectious diseases of the digestive tracts, including giardia (also known as mountain fever or beaver fever), cholera, and dysentery, getting the patient to swallow as much *E. angustifolia* as could be forced down. The digestive infections must be seen in their true context to appreciate these uses of the plant. Mountain fever, cholera and dysentery were potentially terminal diseases, especially for children. The power of *E. angustifolia* to save the lives of children, caused the Eclectic's to pay it particular attention.

Syphilis
Contrary to popular belief, people have always had a lot of sex: the genitals are not a recent source of entertainment. Syphilis was spread through sexual contact, and there was no shortage of syphilis out on the prairie. The Eclectics treated fathers, mothers, and children suffering from syphilis infection. Unlike the bacterial diseases we have looked at so far, this bacterium takes its time to

kill the patient. It starts as a rash, and in time attacks every system in the body, including the brain, heart and bones. Unchecked this disease literally decomposes a person.

Now, *E. angustifolia* had long been used to treat syphilis when Dr Webster started using it, and when his own observations confirmed its value he did not hesitate to advocate its use:

> Dr Goss commends this agent very highly in its treatment of syphilis—in both secondary and tertiary stages. Antisyphilitics are so few, and so unreliable generally, that we may well afford to investigate the merits of this new acquisition, in this direction.

*　　*　　*

Harvey Wickes Felter, MD, *Syllabus of Eclectic Materia Medica and Therapeutics*, compiled from notes taken from the lectures of F. J. Locke, edited with pharmacological additions by H. W. Felter, second edition, Scudder Brothers Company, Cincinnati 1901 Medicinal applications listed in the text:

Acute bacterial infection: diphtheria, septicaemia, spinal meningitis, typhoid fever.

Chronic bacterial infection: tuberculosis, syphilis.

Healing: unhealthful conditions of the mouth and fauces, chronic ulceration.

Dr Felter's guide to the medicinal plants used by the Eclectics extends the applications of *E. angustifolia* and offers some very specific guidance to its use. Here we find a doctor 'in love' with a medicinal plant:

> This remedy is one of the most important of our recent accessions. It is both alterative and antiseptic. It is used in many disorders of the blood, as syphilis, scrofula, and chronic ulcerations. It is one of the reliable remedies for blood poisoning.

49

The fresh root scraped and given freely is the treatment used by the Sioux Indians for snake bite. It is a remedy of some value in typhoid fever, and is well spoken of in diphtheria, spinal meningitis, and in unhealthy conditions of the mouth and fauces ... The dose of this remedy ranges from two to ten drops of the specific preparation.

We have here two additions to our list of bacterial diseases treated by *E. angustifolia*, one acute and one chronic. The first addition, spinal meningitis, is a medical emergency even today. In this acute infection, bacteria move into the meninges, the wrapping of the spinal cord and brain. When bacteria invade the central nervous system serious problems ensue, and may be fatal. It is amazing to discover that the Eclectics found that *E. angustifolia* made a difference in this dreaded disease, which is still a killer today.

The second bacterial disease listed by Dr Felter is tuberculosis, which causes a dangerous condition known as scrofula, also described as end-phase tuberculosis when it enters the lymph nodes, as it often does. The Eclectics found that *E. angustifolia* improved this chronic bacterial infection, and with it the usual course was altered.

Dr Felter also talks about chronic ulceration being treated with *E. angustifolia*. This is very interesting to the student of herbal medicine. Earlier we read that *E. angustifolia* was used when the health failed and the 'natural elements' were moving in for the kill. When people develop chronic ulcers it is a sign that there are some serious problems with their health, and that the body is no longer able to cope. The elderly and those confined to bed often develop these ulcers. Once again, we read that *E. angustifolia* can be used to stimulate a debilitated body to heal itself. Once again, Dr Felter stresses that *E. angustifolia* is the plant to be used:

Specific Echinacea is made of the root gathered in the far West. *(angustifolia)*. This differs materially in properties from that grown farther East. *(purpurea)*. It has but little taste, but leaves in the throat and tongue a tingling sensation.

Echinacea causes an excessive flow of saliva and perspiration.

Another important detail contained here is that *E. angustifolia* doses, properly prepared and medicinally active, should leave a tingly sensation in the mouth. The Eclectics found that when the tingly sensation was present the drug worked, when it was not present, they did not. Some doctors were able to run out and collect their *E. angustifolia* and others had to rely on supply companies. Felter is telling the doctor on the mail order programme that freshness is all-important.

Having warned against *E. purpurea*, Dr Felter is equally dismissive of *E. pallida*. It too lacks the compounds that make the mouth tingle. Two species tossed out in one go! Thank you Dr Felter for answering one of our questions.

*   *   *

F. J. Peterson, MD, *Materia Medica and Clinical Therapeutics*, published by the Author, Los Olivos, California, 1905
Medicinal applications listed in the text:

Acute bacterial infection: appendicitis, diphtheria, cerebrospinal meningitis, cholera infantum, cholera morbus, diarrhoea, erysipelas, gonorrhoea, pneumonia, puerperal fever, septic fevers, septicaemia, septicaemia following abortion, septicaemia following childbirth, tonsillitis, typhoid fever.

Chronic bacterial infection: tuberculosis, acute syphilis, chronic syphilis.

Viral disease: catarrh, measles, nasal catarrh, rabies, smallpox.

Healing: boils, carbuncles, dissecting wounds, inflammation of the male urethra, inflammation of the female urethra, inflammation of the vagina, sores, surgical wounds, ulcers, ulcerated sore throat.

Auto-immune disease: eczema, skin diseases of a systemic origin.

The Eclectic Institute was always located in Ohio, but as more and more graduates passed through its doors, its influence spread far and wide. Dr Peterson was an Eclectic physician who had made it all the way to the West Coast. By now there were thousands of Eclectic doctors around the country, all of them wise to the virtues of *E. angustifolia*. Here is Dr Peterson's verdict on the plant:

> The remedy in all depraved conditions of the blood. Has an alterative and restorative effect on the tissues, hastens retrograde metamorphosis and has marked antiseptic properties; therefore its range of usefulness in both acute and chronic affections is large.

Never were truer words typed. In this text, we find more bacterial and viral diseases being treated with *E. angustifolia*. We also see it being used to heal up surgical wounds, on top of the usual chronic ulcers. Very interestingly, we now find it being used to treat chronic skin diseases like eczema. This is clearly a plant with a wide application.

The key to studying herbal medicine is developing a keen eye for important clues. Dr Peterson calls for the use of *E. angustifolia* 'in good sized doses'—not minute, moderate, or average, but substantial. This is a consistent statement throughout all the Eclectic medical books. If you want to use *E. angustifolia*, you must use it in big doses.

Dr Peterson also brings up a new use of *E. angustifolia*. He says that it can be used in chronic skin conditions. Previously we have read about it being used to treat wounds and sores in people with failing vitality. This is different. Here he talks about using it in diseases like eczema. Eczema is caused by an overly active immune system, a situation in which the immune system overreacts. These conditions are caused by hyper-vitality.

Peterson also leaves us specific instructions recommending that *E. angustifolia* should be used in smaller doses in chronic disease, and larger frequent doses in acute disease. In both cases, a saturated tincture made of the fresh root is recommended. Remember, a saturated tincture is made from one part Echinacea root and one part liquid.

In poisonous bites of rattlesnakes, tarantulas, wasps, etc. give in ¼ to ½ teaspoonful doses every ¼ to ½ hour, until relieved; then in smaller doses and at longer intervals; it should also be applied to the sore pure or in 25 to 50% solution according to the severity of the case. The average dose of Echinacea is from 5 to 10 drops 3 to 4 times a day; but in severe cases and poisoning of the blood by poisonous bites, etc., it must be used in much larger doses and at short intervals. Locally use pure or in 25 to 50% solution.

*   *   *

A. F. Stephens, MD, *The Essentials of Medical Gynecology*, Scudder Brothers Company, Cincinnati 1907
As the Eclectic movement went on, the medical reformers became specialised in fields such as gynaecology and paediatrics. In the medical books they published on specific subjects, *E. angustifolia* surfaces consistently for a variety of purposes.

Women have always resorted to abortions, and in the days before it was legal this led to disastrous results. Countless women have died from bad abortions, frequently because bacteria have spread to the uterus, bringing a lethal infection. *E. angustifolia* was used to save women who had suffered a bad abortion. Dr Stephens recommends it whenever gynaecological infection sets in. This is an important note, because these infections are still causing problems today.

*   *   *

Harvey Wickes Felter, *King's American Dispensatory*, Ohio Valley Company, Cincinnati, Ohio, 1909
Medicinal applications listed in the text:

Acute bacterial infection: systemic infections, puerperal fever, septicaemia, scarlet fever.

Infections of the digestive tract: cholera infantum, cholera morbus, diphtheria, diarrhoea, dysentery, perityphilitis, typhoid, typho-malaria, typhilitis.

Infections of the throat: quinsy, streptococcal infection, tonsillitis.

Infections of the reproductive tract: gonorrhoea, inflammation of gonorrhoea, painful mammitis, leucorrhea, leucorrhea with offensive discharge, ulceration of the os uteri, purulent salpingitis, erythematous or erysipelatous vulvitis.

Infections of the respiratory tract: ulcerated and fetid mucous surfaces with dusky or dark coloration, general debilitated constitution, catarrhal affections of the nasopharynx and nose, catarrhal affections of the respiratory tract, fetid bronchitis, pulmonary gangrene, typhoid pneumonia, tubercular abscesses, empyema with gangrene.

Infections of the skin: erysipelas with sloughing phagenia.

Chronic bacterial infection: syphilis, syphilitic ulcers of mouth, throat and tongue, tuberculosis, tubercular diathesis, tubercular phthisis.

Viral infection: chicken-pox, epidemic influenza, influenza, measles, rabies, smallpox.

Protozoal infection: acute malaria, chronic malaria, giardia.

Poisoning: stings of wasps and bees with painful swelling, rattle-snake bite, tarantula bite.

Healing: digestive system, fermentative dyspepsia, offensive breath, duodenal catarrh, intestinal indigestion with pain and debility, ulcerative stomatitis, nursing sore mouth, dyspepsia.

*Skin:*phlegmonous swellings, old sores, dissecting wounds, surgical wounds, dermatitis venenata, pus-filled cavities, abscesses, malignant carbuncles, chronic leg ulcers, painful chronic eruptions, chronic ulcers, gangrene.

Auto-immune disease: corneal ulcers, chronic eczema with sticky or glutinous exudation, eczema, eczematous eruptions, iritis, psoriasis, rheumatism, scarlet fever leading to angina and rheumatic attacks.

Cancer: cancerous growths, cancer of the mucous membrane, cancer of the fauces, odour of carcinoma, mammary cancer, cancerous cachexia, testicular cancer.

In 1909, the Eclectic Bible, *King's Dispensatory*, was re-released. The prominent Eclectic, Dr Felter, revised the original text to include the discoveries made in the fifty-six years that had passed since King first wrote his dispensatory. If you compare the list of uses for *E. angustifolia* in the original book with those mentioned in this new and improved version, it is clear that the Eclectics had learned a fair amount over the years! The uses of the plant had multiplied dramatically. What we have here is a window on the world of *Echinacea angustifolia* at the turn of the century, an informed summary of all that the Eclectics had learned about the plant.

Working in the field of herbal medicine, I am forever being told that the subject has not been properly studied. I beg to differ. Compare the first *King's Dispensatory* with the second, and you recognise how thoroughly the Eclectics had studied *E. angustifolia*. Here we see a long list of appropriate uses. What we don't see is all the uses *rejected* by the Eclectics—rejected because they found they did not work!

Remember that the Eclectics were shunned by the regular medical profession from the word go. At first it was because they contradicted the medical establishment, but as the Eclectics became known for their ability to cure infectious disease, matters only got worse. The Eclectics had an 80–90 per cent cure rate for infectious disease prior to the age of antibiotics. The orthodox physicians had a 20 per cent cure rate. This ability to cure the 'incurable' made the Eclectics popular with the people and hated by the ordinary doctors. There was no spirit of cooperation between these rival schools.

Orthodox physicians initially rejected *E. angustifolia* out of hand; they said it was more Eclectic lunacy. Even when the Eclectics could show success with it, the orthodox group stuck with their opinion. Professional pride came first. But the time came when they could not look the other way. They had no choice but to start using *E. angustifolia*. At this point it was the Eclectics who felt threatened. They were terrified that their rivals would steal their glory. Hence Dr Felter's proud claim:

Conspicuous among the remedies introduced within recent years, Echinacea (*angustifolia*) undoubtedly takes the first rank.

Though now a well-known drug, [the plant] stands peculiarly alone in being essentially a new remedy. Many remedies which have lately been introduced, can be traced back for years, and some of them for centuries, as having at some time occupied a place in either domestic or professional practice, but our ancient scientific works are silent concerning this species of Echinacea. A careful search through the large numbers of works upon domestic medicine, herbal, medical botanies, and the so-called 'irregular' works upon practice, contained in the Lloyd Library, failed to reveal even a mention of *Echinacea angustifolia* as a medicinal agent. The first notices concerning Echinacea (*angustifolia*) are from Eclectic physicians, and the drug is, from start to finish, an Eclectic medicine.

Dr Felter had set the record straight. (Note that he does not mention the Native American connection.) He was also at pains to focus his readers' attention by giving details enabling them to identify and use the correct species:

Echinacea angustifolia is an indigenous plant of the composite, growing chiefly in the Western states, from Illinois to Nebraska, and Southward through Missouri to Texas, thriving best in rich prairie soil. That which grows in marshy places is of inferior quality ... The plant blooms from June to August ...

The scientific appellations are derived from physical features of the plant, and are therefore descriptive. The generic term *Echinacea*, is derived from the Greek *echinos*, meaning hedge-hog or sea-urchin, referring to the spiny, hedge-hog like fruiting head; while the specific name *angustifolia*, comes from the two Latin words, *angustus* (narrow) and *folium* (leaf), contrasting thereby this species with the other forms of Echinacea, this being the narrow-leaved species.

This is still more conclusive proof that those who invoke the Eclectics in connection with the other two species of Echinacea are misguided when they do so. The Eclectics wanted nothing to do with either *E. purpurea* or *E. pallida*, and there is no disputing this fact.

The search and research process
There are those in the scientific community who view herbal medicines with suspicion and severe scepticism. This crew of doubters loves to run herbal medicines into the ground by saying that there is no clinical trial evidence that they work. Their statements betray their ignorance. Dr Felter's account makes it clear that the Eclectics first viewed *E. angustifolia* with suspicion, and only after extensive trials did they become convinced of its efficacy. He mentions a whole series of authorities, and trials that went back for half a century. I don't think the same could be said for drugs like Prozac, which oddly enough do have the blessing of the scientific community. The striking fact is that *E. angustifolia* passed the scientific test long before the current critics of herbal medicine were born!

At the same time, the Eclectic's found themselves astonished by the sheer range of application of the plant. In those days drugs were classified according to their action. In the case of *E. angustifolia*, the problem was to put it into a pigeon hole; it simply did too many things to be categorised. In the next lines we see evidence of the Eclectic struggle to put a label on this extraordinary medicinal substance:

Under the older classification of remedies, Echinacea would probably be classed as an antiseptic and alterative. Strictly speaking, it is practically impossible to classify an agent like Echinacea by applying to it one or two words to indicate its virtues. The day is rapidly approaching when these qualifying claims will have no place in medicine, for they but inadequately convey to our minds, the therapeutic possibilities of our drugs.

Especially is this so with regard to such terms as alterative, stimulant, tonic, etc. If any single statement were to be made concerning the virtues of Echinacea, it would read something like this: A corrector of the depravation of the body fluids, and even this does not sufficiently cover the ground. Its extraordinary powers, combining essentially that formerly included under the terms antiseptic, antifermentative, and antizymotic are well shown in its power over changes produced in the fluids of the body, whether from internal causes or from external introductions.

The changes may be manifested in a disturbed balance of the fluids resulting in such tissue alterations as are exhibited in boils, carbuncles, abscesses, or cellular glandular inflammations. They may be from the introduction of serpent or insect venom, or they may be due to such fearful poisons as give rise to malignant diphtheria, cerebrospinal meningitis, or puerperal and other forms of septicaemia.

Such changes, whether they be septic or of devitalized morbid accumulations, or alterations in the fluids themselves, appear to have met their antagonist in Echinacea. 'Bad blood', so called asthenia, or adynamia, and particularly a tendency to malignancy in acute and sub-acute disorders, seem to be special indicators for the use of Echinacea.

The Eclectics knew that *E. angustifolia* did something that affected a wide range of diseases, but they were not certain what that was, so they could not account for its activity. However, while they puzzled over its means of operation they kept on using it and learning more and more about its activity in disease. Dr Felter's text reveals the turn-of-the-century uses of *E. angustifolia* in far more detail than we have space to reproduce. We will pick out just a few points that stand out from our present-day perspective, using a century's hindsight.

Cancer. The Eclectics took the view that cancer only developed in people whose health was failing. Today we know that the immune system is responsible for killing cancer cells, and when the immune system fails, cancer cells do indeed have the opportunity to grow unmolested. In this text we see the Eclectics homing in on the type of person likely to develop cancer. They considered that *E. angustifolia* was excellent for those with a 'tendency to malignancy', a tendency to cancer:

> It is reported to have relieved the pain of cancerous growths, particularly when involving the mucous membranes, as cancer of the fauces. Prof. Farnum calls attention to the wonderful rapidity with which the odour of carcinoma is overcome by echafolta. He strongly recommends it as an application for cancer, and relates a case of mammary cancer long held in check by it. He also advises its internal administration in cancerous cachexia.

Slow-healing wounds. When a body is falling apart, it lacks vitality to heal wounds. The elderly, confined to bed, often develop bed sores which simply will not heal. Indeed the elderly not confined to bed often develop varicose ulcers that simply will not knit together. *E. angustifolia* was prescribed in all of these cases.

Auto-immune diseases. In this text we have seen mention of diseases of an auto-immune origin, that is diseases in which the problem rests with the immune system attacking the body. Commonly known auto-immune diseases are allergies, rheumatoid arthritis and eczema. These diseases fall into the 'from within' category, as the problem lies with an over-active immune system. Sometimes these conditions are described as hyper-immune disease, as the immune system functions in an overzealous manner.

Digestive disturbances. When the immune system goes wrong and starts attacking itself, the entire body becomes fair game for attack. The skin, the joints, the respiratory tract and the digestive tract often become targets for immune system abuse. In this text we find that the Eclectics recommend *E. angustifolia* for the auto-immune diseases affecting the digestive tract:

> Echinacea is a good appetizer, and improves digestion. The writer has used it with good results in fermentative dyspepsia, with offensive breath and gastric pain as prominent symptoms, which was also aggravated upon taking food. It is also efficient in duodenal catarrh, and other forms of intestinal indigestion, with pain and debility. Few remedies are as efficient in ulcerative stomatitis, and in nursing sore-mouth it is asserted to be promptly curative.

Bacterial infection. The Eclectics used Echinacea in a wide host of acute bacterial infections, whether the bacteria was in the blood, in the tonsils, or in the uterus. Bacterial infection is once again a major issue, and we need to take note that *E. angustifolia* can be of use in these conditions. The ugly words 'antibiotic-resistant strain' spring to mind. Septicaemia—bacteria in the blood—and meningitis—bacteria in the brain—are two very dangerous conditions that this plant proved able to treat.

Chronic bacterial infection. There are some bacterial infections which take their time killing off the person, the two most notable being syphilis and tuberculosis. In both cases, the Eclectics found that *E. angustifolia* kept the condition under control. There is no shortage of antibiotic-resistant tuberculosis and syphilis about today, making these important lines. If antibiotics don't do the job, then *E. angustifolia* might!

Viral disease. The Eclectics used *E. angustifolia* in viral disease from the beginning. However, what they said about it in these cases is important. When it was administered the conditions that usually followed on—as in pneumonia after influenza—did not occur. Viral disease poses a great threat today, and the following lines may spark the imagination of those working on the front line of health care.

In the eruptive fevers, as measles, chicken-pox, and scarlet fever, [Echinacea] has received some praise, especially for its control over the catarrhal phases of the former. Like many other new remedies Echinacea has been reported curative in smallpox.

Epidemic influenza (la grippe) is occasionally ameliorated by Echinacea, and in all such cases, with great debility, it assists materially in securing a good convalescence.

Likewise Echinacea has been recommended to prevent hydrophobia. How one can prevent a result of this kind from a dog bite, and especially as the very existence of that so-called disease is denied by many is not clear.

Protozoal infection. Much like bacteria, malaria has become resistant to many of the drugs used today. The following lines suggest that *E. angustifolia* might be a powerful addition to the anti-malaria effort:

Notwithstanding that it has been recommended as one of the best antimalarial remedies, it appears to exert but little influence over periodicity. Prof. King reported signal failure in every case of ague in which he gave it a trial. Others, however, speak of it as a remedy for malaria when of an asthenic character. Possibly in such conditions it might prove of value, as the fevers in which it has proved so successful have been chiefly characterized by adynamia. Very likely its usefulness here depends more upon its influence over the asthenia than upon the miasmatic poison. However, Dr. Snyder . . . , a good authority, contends that it is an excellent remedy for chronic malaria, a personal use of it having first convinced him of its value.

Dosage and frequency

As the Eclectics were the masters of *E. angustifolia*, the manner in which they used the medicine is very important. We have learned the conditions in which they felt it was helpful, now we can focus briefly on how they used it. The updated *King's Dispensatory* leaves us with the true cutting edge of *E. angustifolia* use. As we have learned, the Eclectics used it in large doses. In this text we also find it recommended in large doses, but we see something else: that the medicine was best administered frequently—especially in acute infections. Dr Felter tells us that it should be used every half an hour, and he meant around the clock. Large and frequent doses is the message.

*   *   *

John Williams Fyfe, MD, *Pocket Essentials of Modern Materia Medica and Therapeutics*, Scudder Brothers Company, 1911
Medicinal applications listed in the text:

Acute bacterial infection: cholera infantum, diphtheria, erysipelas, scarlet fever, spinal meningitis, typhoid fever, typhoid pneumonia.

Chronic bacterial infection: remittent and intermittent fevers, syphilis, tuberculosis.

Viral disease: cerebrospinal meningitis, rabies.

Healing: old sores, old wounds, tendency to boils and carbuncles.

Poisoning: poisonous stings, snakebite.

Dr Fyfe, unlike the earlier Eclectics, kept his comments about medicinal plants brief and to the point! To a large extent, we see much of the same material that we have seen before. *E. angustifolia* is a powerful tool against poisoning, from within and from without. Cholera, diphtheria, rabies and slow-healing wounds are once again found to be effectively treated with the plant.

Waste removal. In his first paragraph Dr Fyfe introduces an important activity of *E. angustifolia*. When a person has a bacterial infection, an infected wound, or has been bitten by a venomous animal, tissue is killed by the offending agents, whether bacteria or venom. The body has to move this dead tissue out of the system. Dr Fyfe indicates that *E. angustifolia* speeds the removal of dead tissue, thus facilitating the healing process. This has been inferred by earlier Eclectics, but never articulated so well. He finds it effective in cases of:

Tongue coated black, putrescent odour from excess of broken down material being eliminated from the system, as in scarlet fever, diphtheria, spinal meningitis and typhoid fever, strumous diathesis, old sores and wounds, snake bites and bites of rabid dogs, tendency to boils and carbuncles.

Most modern medical professionals are consumed with the acute phase of an illness, say the period of time when streptococci are making a mess of the tonsils, or when the influenza virus is wreaking havoc. However the convalescent period is just as important and needs equal attention. Acute illness causes damage to the body that needs cleaning up. Like a battlefield after the battle, the body can be a mess after the infection has been conquered. The immune system is responsible for conquering the enemy and cleaning up the post-battle mess. The Eclectics tell us not to forget *E. angustifolia* in the restorative phase.

* * *

Finley Ellingwood, MD, *American Materia Medica, Therapeutics, and Pharmacognosy*, Ellingwood's Therapeutist, Chicago 1919
Medicinal applications in the text:

Acute bacterial infections: anthrax, cerebrospinal meningitis, cholera infantum, cholera morbus, diphtheria, erysipelas, general infection following vaccinations, gonorrhoea, leucorrhea, mastitis, puerperal fever, puerperal sepsis, pyemia, septicaemia, septic fever, tetanus, typhoid, typhoid fever.

Chronic bacterial infections: syphilis, syphilitic nodules, stubborn skin conditions associated with syphilis, tuberculosis, tubercular nodules.

Viral infections: fever sores, rabies, smallpox.

Protozoal infections: malaria, malarial fevers.

Fungal infections: actinomycosis, impetigo contagioso.

Poisoning: snakebite, tarantula bite, scorpion bite, strychnine poisoning.

Cancer: breast cancer, cancer in general.

Healing: tendency to gangrenous states, boils, carbuncles, abscesses, abscesses of the sinuses, cellular and glandular abscesses, inflammation of any portion of the intestine, chronic inflammation of the breast, wounds, bed sores, fever sores, ulcerated mouth, ulcerated throat, ulcerated post nasal passages, ulceration of tibial surfaces (chronic), ulceration of glandular tissues, gangrene, nettle rash, piles.

Auto-immune diseases: anaemia, glandular ulcerations, chronic skin diseases, skin disorders, psoriasis, eruptive skin diseases with purulent discharge, hyperthyroid disease, ulcerative colitis, diabetes mellitus, diabetes insipidus, albuminuria, alopecia.

After a long journey through the Eclectic use of *E. angustifolia*, we have reached our final text. Shortly after this textbook was published, the Eclectic Institute closed its doors. After eighty years of trying, the orthodox physicians had finally succeeded in running them out of business. With the school gone there was no need for textbooks. It was the end of the road for the long relationship between the Eclectics and *Echinacea angustifolia*. However, this final text provides us with an authoritative summary of the Eclectics' findings about the plant, and a last opportunity to hear what the masters had to say.

Dr Ellingwood starts his text with his general opinion of *E. angustifolia*. To put this in perspective, the Eclectics were a cantankerous group. They fought with each other continuously and agreed upon very few points. At times their disagreements turned so nasty that there are accounts of them pulling guns at board meetings. Yet on the virtues of *E. angustifolia* no battles were fought. Those who agreed upon little were united over this medicinal plant:

> For from twenty to twenty-five years, Echinacea has been passing through the stages of critical experimentation under the observation of several thousand physicians, and its remarkable properties are receiving positive confirmation. As yet, but few disparaging statements have been made. All who use it correctly fall quickly into line as enthusiasts in its praise; the experience of the writer is similar to that of the rest, the results in nearly all cases having been satisfactory. The laboratory observations have been extensive but are not yet complete.

The Eclectics closed the Institute's doors as firm supporters of *E. angustifolia*. To them it was an excellent medicine which had saved thousands of people's lives and pulled innumerable patients back from the brink of death. We shall sample some of the practical experience summed up by Dr Ellingwood, starting with this key reminder, which is basic to the Eclectics' approach:

> There is considerable confusion concerning the identity of the active medicinal species of echinacea. The *Echinacea purpurea* of the Eastern States has been thought to be identical with the *Echinacea angustifolia* of the Western States. It is often used for the same purposes, but is universally disappointing.

Dr Ellingwood is categorical here. *E. purpurea*, in his experience, was 'disappointing'—not occasionally or intermittently, but *universally* disappointing. To him, as to all the Eclectics, there was only one Echinacea species to use, and that species was *E. angustifolia*.

Poison in the blood

It is the remedy for blood poisoning, if there is one in the
Materia Medica. Its field covers acute auto-infection, slow
progressive blood taint, faults of the blood from imperfect
elimination of all possible character, and from the development of disease germs within the blood.

Regardless of the source of poisoning, whether caused by the body
or by an organism taking the body hostage, *E. angustifolia* was the
drug. Ellingwood gives us three examples of poisoning. It could be
injected into the body, as in the case of a venomous snake bite. It
could be produced by bacteria having taken up residence in the body.
Or it could be the poison produced by the body itself, auto-
intoxication as Dr Ellingwood puts it—today we would call this an
auto-immune disease. Ellingwood indicates that 'poison' in the
system will manifest itself differently in different people. Regardless
of how it does so, whether it be in the skin or in nervous system
irregularities, *E. angustifolia* will address the fundamental problem.

It acts equally well, whether the profound influence be exerted
upon the nervous system, as in puerperal sepsis, and uraemia,
or whether there be prostration and exhaustion, as in perni-
cious malarial and septic fevers or whether its influence is
shown by anaemia, glandular ulceration or skin disease.

In earlier texts we found that *E. angustifolia* was specifically of
use when the body was prone to infection, unable to fight off the
elements, and approaching a state of degeneration. Ellingwood adds:

It is especially indicated where there is a tendency to gangrenous states and sloughing of the soft tissue, throat dark and
full, tongue full, with dirty dark-brown or black coat, in all
cases where there are sepsis and zymosis.

Broadly speaking, then, *E. angustifolia* should be used when
the body was failing, whether due to internal or external causes!

How does Echinacea work?

In Dr Ellingwood's text we find a really exciting development. At this time the Eclectics were working in the laboratory to figure out how *E. angustifolia* worked. The result was that they tracked down the source of its special magic.

For the sake of the non-medical reader, a quick review of the immune system will be helpful. First of all, the immune system is comprised of cells, that float around in the blood looking for bacteria, virus, and cancer cells that need killing. These wandering hunters are known as white blood cells. When the early microscopists looked at human blood, they noticed that it contained two types of cell, red and white. The white ones were dubbed 'leucocytes'—'white-cells' in Greek. In time the early workers noticed that there were different types of leucocytes, and they each were given a different name, depending on what they did or how they looked. The early workers discovered that white blood cells roamed the body hoovering up bacteria and destroying them.

In the following text we see that the Eclectics had discovered that *E. angustifolia* worked by increasing the number of white blood cells and stimulating these cells to increased activity. It was an immune stimulant. These tests were not conducted on lab animals, they were conducted on patients hospitalised and under the care of Eclectic physicians. This text is vitally important to the *E. angustifolia* story. Helpful translations for the non-medical person have been added.

Physiological Action—The following laboratory observations of its action upon the blood were made by Victor von Unruh, M.D., of New York City: more than one hundred blood counts were made in cases of infectious diseases, mainly in tuberculosis. 'The results showed that Echinacea increases the phagocytic power of the leucocytes; it normalizes the percentage count of the neutrophiles (Arneth count).'

(A phagocyte is a cell that has the power to consume foreign material. When *E. angustifolia* was administered to patients, their white blood cells were better able to kill bacteria.)

> The stimulation toward phagocytosis became very evident in cases where it was impossible to find any evidence of phagocytosis before *Echinacea angustifolia* was administered, and where after the use of this drug for a period of only a few days, the phagocytes were seen to contain as many as eight bacilli within the cell. In all cases where the percentage count among the neutrophiles (polymorphonuclears) has been such as to give an unfavourable prognosis ... the administration of Echinacea for only two weeks has normalized the percentage ... Echinacea thus gives to the class normally strongest in phagocytosis the power where it obtains in the normal condition of the leucocytes.

(In patients who had low white blood cells, when *E. angustifolia* was administered, they quickly had lots more white blood cells out there hoovering up bacteria. *E. angustifolia* increased the number of white blood cells.)

For nearly seventy years, the Eclectics had insisted that *E. angustifolia* cured bacterial infection. They did not know how it did it, but they suspected it worked on the blood. At long last, as science progressed, it found the explanation. *E. angustifolia* increased the number of bacterial-killing white blood cells, and the rate at which they worked.

In a related context, we see the degree to which the Eclectics were living before their time. Quite recently we have learned that the body produces substances—interferon is an example—which turn on the immune system. These substances are called 'cellular mediators' and they are signals to the immune system to get busy. Ellingwood suggests that *E. angustifolia* improved the immune system, by prompting the body to produce substances that stimulated that system:

> I have long been assured from the observation of this remedy that it directly influences the opsonic index. I wrote von

Unruh directly, asking him for his opinion from his long experience and from his laboratory observations of the action of this remedy. He replied as follows: 'Quoting from McFarland's *Pathogenic Bacteria*, the opsonic theory teaches that the leucocytes are disinclined to take up bacteria unless they are prepared for phagocytosis by contact with certain substances in the serum, that in some manner modify them. This modifying substance is the opsonin. I have definitely demonstrated and am continuing to observe, that the action of Echinacea on the leucocytes is such that it will raise phagocytosis to its possible maximum. The logical deduction, therefore, is that the opsonic index is correspondingly raised by this agent.'

Before the Eclectics called it quits, they found their explanation as to why *E. angustifolia* helped some people to survive infection and helped others avoid infection in the first place. The key to all of its activities was immune system activation. Before we leave this discovery section, we must look at another quote, which deals with a different kind of problem with this system. Leukaemia, a fatal disease, is caused by a rapid and dangerous increase in white blood cell count. For reasons that still elude scientists today, the immune system starts producing more white blood cells than red blood cells. Too much of a good thing is as bad as too little. When the body produces this massive quantity of white blood cells, it does so in a sloppy manner—the cells are very immature in appearance. As you will see, the Eclectics found that in dealing with leukaemia, *E. angustifolia* corrected the balance of red to white blood cells:

Hyperleukocytosis and leucopenia are directly improved by Echinacea; the proportion of white to red cells is rendered normal; and the elimination of waste products is stimulated to a degree which puts this drug in the first rank among all alteratives.

(When white blood cell counts were excessively high, adminis-

69

tering *E. angustifolia* would result in a normalisation of the blood cell count.)

The Eclectics discovered that *E. angustifolia* normalised immune system function, whether it was too low or too high. Here we see how they observed this on a cellular level, having already observed it on a clinical level. This raises some serious questions and is very thought-provoking.

A non-toxic treatment

Wooster Beach started the Eclectic movement because he could not abide the dangerous and toxic medicines being used by the 'regulars' of his day. The Eclectics felt that medicine should be non-toxic and non-injurious to the body, and whenever they worked with a medicine they conducted experiments to make certain that it did no harm. More often than not they used themselves as guinea pigs. One doctor would ingest a huge quantity of the medicine, and another would watch to see what happened. This was rough and ready science! The following lines describe the effects of such an intentional overdose of *E. angustifolia*:

> The toxic effect of this agent is manifested by reduction of temperature, the frequency of the pulse is diminished, the mucous membrane becomes dry and parched, accompanied with a prickly sensation; there is headache of a bursting character, and a tendency to fainting is observed if the patient assumes an erect posture. After poisonous doses, these symptoms are more intensified. The face and upper portion of the trunk are flushed, there is pain throughout the body, which is more marked in the large articulations. There is dimness of vision, intense thirst, gastric pains followed by vomiting and watery diarrhoea. No fatal case of poisoning is recorded, to our knowledge, and only when given in extreme doses are any of the above undesirable influences observed. There are but few subjective symptoms from large doses of this agent. It is apparently non-toxic, and to any unpleasant extent non-irritant.

The Eclectics advocated using *E. angustifolia* in large and frequent amounts, but first they overdosed themselves time and time again to make certain that the plant was non-toxic. Most of them lived a long life—proof positive that it was safe.

Bacterial infection

The Eclectics found that all bacterial infections were fair game for *E. angustifolia*. This is important to know, because we in the modern age are confronting bacterial disease which will not yield to antibiotics. The term 'antibiotic-resistant strain' is commonplace, because killer bugs are at large. We need to look closely at the Eclectic use of *E. angustifolia* in bacterial disease, because one day we might face a situation where a non-antibiotic alternative will keep us or one of our loved ones alive.

Ellingwood knew that the problem with bacterial infection was not the bacteria, but rather the toxins they produced. The toxins produced by typhoid attacked the nervous system; those of diphtheria destroyed the tissue of the digestive tract. They found that in bacterial infection, tissue was not destroyed when *E. angustifolia* was employed. This plant would act against toxins, whether produced by bacteria or by serpents.

> Echinacea is par excellence a corrector of any depravation of the body fluids. It influences those conditions included under the terms septic, fermentative and zymotic. Those which manifest themselves in a disturbed balance of the fluids, resulting in alterations of the tissues such as are exhibited in boils, carbuncles, abscesses and cellular and glandular inflammations. These same conditions result from the introduction of the venom of serpents and poisonous insects of every character, also from the introduction of disease germs from pus and other putrid and infectious sources.

The Eclectics also knew that the presence of bacteria caused a fever response from the body: it heated up to 'incinerate' the bacteria. Unfortunately, the brain and other important body bits could get singed in the process. Controlling temperature while the immune system was dealing with the bacteria was critical if the patient was to survive. They found that when *E. angustifolia* was administered, temperatures came down:

> In several cases reported, the temperature has declined from one-half to two degrees within a few hours after its use was begun, and has not increased until the agent was discontinued. It has then slowly increased toward the previous high point until the remedy was again taken, when a decline was soon apparent.
>
> It does not produce abrupt drops in the temperature ... but it effects an almost immediate stop in germ development, and a steady restoration from its pernicious influence. In the treatment of typhoid fever in the Cook County Hospital, Chicago, it was used in the Eclectic wards for about two years, or more, and twenty-one days was the extreme extent of the fever, and the mortality was the lowest known. In many cases taken early, the fever was limited to fourteen days without delirium. In private practice the reports of many physicians are much more enthusiastic, claiming that when given in the initial stage, the fever has disappeared in seven days, and that fourteen days is the extreme limit.

Let's take a final look at the bacterial and viral infections treated with *Echinacea angustifolia*. Remember, you may need this information one day.

Diphtheria

> It has been in constant use in diphtheria for three years. It is used locally as well as internally. The exudates contract and disappear, the local evidences of septic absorption are gone, the fever declines, the vital forces increase, depression, mental and physical disappears, and the improvement is continual.
>
> Dr. Fair is emphatic in his statements that patients exposed to diphtheria should take Echinacea in from ten to twenty drop doses every two hours with the positive expectation of

preventing the disease. If the first symptoms appear as the usual premonitory evidences, the dose should be increased and other indicated remedies will ward off the disease. I have much confidence in this statement and would suggest that it be carried out fully.

Cholera

Its use in cholera infantum has been satisfactory, especially if nervous phenomena are present. The frequent discharges gradually cease, the patient is soothed and the nerve force increases as the fever abates. Extreme nervous phenomena do not appear.

Spinal meningitis

Webster, of San Francisco, in 1892, suggested the use of Echinacea in spinal meningitis. It should be especially valuable if any blood dyscrasia lies at the bottom of the difficulty. Following Webster's suggestions, other physicians, from their personal observations, have been able to ascribe undoubted curative virtues to this agent in this and other convulsive and inflammatory disorders of the brain and cord. It directly antidotes the infection.

Since the above was first written the use of Echinacea for cerebro-spinal meningitis has been established among those who have been experimenting with the remedy. There is no doubt whatever that its influence in destroying the virus is specific, and effectual if given in sufficient doses. Five drops is about the ordinary dose for a child, but this can be increased to twenty in extreme cases.

Erysipelas

In the treatment of erysipelas it has given more than ordinary satisfaction ... It is especially needed when sloughing and tissue disintegration occur, its external influence being most reliable. In the treatment of erysipelas, the remedy has proven itself all we anticipated for it.

Tetanus

A large amount of satisfactory evidence has accumulated confirmatory of our statements concerning the curative action of the remedy in tetanus. Dr. John Herring reported one marked cure. Dr. Lewis reports three cases, where the remedy was injected into the wound after tetanic symptoms had shown themselves. All the tissues surrounding the wound were filled with the remedy by hypodermic injection and gauze saturated with a full strength preparation was kept constantly applied. The agent was also administered in half-dram doses internally, every two or three hours.

Anthrax

In the treatment of Anthrax, Echinacea has proven in a number of cases to be an exceedingly reliable remedy. Dr. Lewis of Canton, Pa., first reported on it in 1907 in Ellingwood's Therapeutist, and Dr. Aylesworth of Collingwood, Canada, confirmed all of his statements, the observations of the two doctors having been made about the same time, each without knowledge of the other. In these cases, very large doses from one to two drams, frequently repeated, are required.

Actinomycosis

Twenty to forty minims of Echinacea every two hours with proper local treatment, such as iodine locally, will cure actinomycosis.

Impetigo

The use of *Echinacea angustifolia* in the treatment of impetigo contagiosa is confirmed. One doctor treated several very severe cases and the rational action of the remedy suggests that its use externally and internally in this disease will prove highly satisfactory.

Urethritis

Another physician whose name is not given, treated infection and a purulent discharge from the urethra where there was urinary retention for two days, with this remedy. He passed a catheter as far down as possible, and then combined one part Echinacea with six parts of sterilized water. He forced this slowly against the constriction. Relaxation took place probably from the local anaesthetic influence of the remedy in a few minutes. The catheter was withdrawn, and the water passed freely. He repeated the treatment once or twice a day to a complete cure.

Appendicitis

In local inflammation of any portion of the intestinal tract, it has given excellent satisfaction. It quickly overcomes local blood stasis, prevents or cures ulceration, and retards pus formation by determining resolution. Reports of its use in appendicitis have been satisfactory, indeed. One writer treated several cases of unmistakable diagnosis, and satisfactory cure resulted. The writer treated one marked case of appendicitis where pus formation and future operation seemed inevitable. The improvement was apparent after the agent had been taken in a few hours, and recovery was complete in twelve days from attack.

Syphilis

In the treatment of syphilis very many observations have been reported. It has been used entirely alone and also in conjunction with alterative syrups, but in no case yet reported has mercury been used with it. The longest time of all cases yet reported, needed to perfect the cure, was nine months.

Rabies

By far the most difficult reports to credit are those of the individuals bitten by rabid animals; there are between twenty and thirty reports at the present time. In no case has hydrophobia yet occurred, and this was the only remedy used in many of the cases. In five or six cases, animals bitten at the same time as the patient had developed rabies, and had even conveyed it to other animals, and yet the patient showed no evidence of poisoning, if the remedy was used at once. One case exhibited the developing symptoms of hydrophobia before the agent was begun. They disappeared shortly after treatment. In no case has an opportunity offered to try the remedy after the symptoms were actually developed.

This account is interesting because, more than using *E. angustifolia* to treat rabies, the Eclectics used it to prevent the disease from setting in. The rabies virus is passed from an infected animal. Once the virus is in the human body, one of two things happens. Either the immune system kills the virus or the virus takes root. If the immune system is all fired up, the rabies has less chance to settle. The Eclectics found that a person bitten by a mad dog and treated with *E. angustifolia* did not develop the disease. This fits the pattern of our knowledge.

Influenza

The Eclectics' opinion on viral infection was that *E. angustifolia* didn't necessarily make the viral disease go away, but the side-effects of viral disease were reduced when it was used. An example in the case of influenza. Those who were treated with the plant did not come down with the secondary infections usually associated with the flu. When people get influenza, they start producing loads of mucus. Mucus creates the ideal environment for bacteria to flourish, so influenza is often followed by pneumonia, tonsillitis, bronchitis, sinusitis, etc. The Eclectics found that all of these follow-ons, or sequelae, were avoided when *E. angustifolia* was used. As they put it, viral disease remained uncomplicated.

Other applications

Poisoning

The Eclectic adventure with *E. angustifolia* started with old Dr Meyer and his rattlesnakes, and Ellingwood approves his predecessor. By now, the Eclectics had discovered that the white blood cells responsible for ingesting bacteria would also ingest poisons such as snakebite venom. Ellingwood also makes one interesting addition to the kinds of poisoning for which *E. angustifolia* is recommended. Up to this point it had been used in natural poisoning, if you will. In these lines the cause is anything but natural:

One doctor had an opportunity to observe the action of Echinacea in some fowl that had taken strychnine which was used to poison animals. Those that received the medicine, lived. All those that did not get it, died.'

The immune cells are responsible for hoovering up toxins, and strychnine would fall into this category. Even when the Eclectics were getting ready to pack it in, they were still experimenting!

Cancer

One of the modern uses of *E. angustifolia* is in the treatment of cancer. Ellingwood reports on a limited use of Echinacea here. Many of the Eclectics used it to clean up the messy sores associated with the spread of cancer and to remove the 'odour of cancer'.

In the pain of mammary cancer and in the chronic inflammation of the mammary gland, the result of badly treated puerperal mastitis, where the part has become reddened and congested, the remedy has worked satisfactorily.

Beyond cleaning out nasty cancerous sores, Echinacea was starting to be used in cancer in general. The following text hints that the Eclectics were starting to see another use for *E. angustifolia*.

Prof. Farnum is enthusiastic over the action of the remedy in overcoming the odour of cancer, whether in the early stages, or in the latter stage of the development of this serious disease. He advises its persistent administration in all cases where there is a cancerous cachexia, believing that it retards the development of cancer and greatly prolongs the patient's life.

Unfortunately, just as the Eclectics started looking at *E. angustifolia*'s effect on cancer, the movement came to an end. Had they gone on for another thirty years, who knows what they would have found? The white blood cells responsible for doing battle with bacteria also tackle cancer cells. The improvement they saw may reflect this same activity.

Healing
The immune cells are not only responsible for killing bacteria and cancer cells, they are also responsible for healing on a fundamental level. Some immune cells clean out dead tissue and others stimulate the formation of granulation tissue, which bridges the gaps in broken tissue. Not only does the immune system keep the body free of 'bad guys', it is also responsible for the healing process. It literally knits things together, when they are broken. The Eclectics had proved that *E. angustifolia* was effective in speeding the healing process and that it was an immune stimulant. Wonder no more why bed-sores disappeared, or why the plant was so effective in treating chronic ulceration, old sores and all kinds of wounds, as well as in cases of gangrene and erysipelas.

Hyper-immune disease

Medicinal plants often have contradictory activities, and those of us who study them have grown accustomed to this. To the inexperienced and the conventionally trained, this can be quite perplexing and at least confusing. In this section, we will learn that the Eclectics used *E. angustifolia* to treat conditions caused, not by poor immune function, but rather by an over-active immune system: conditions we now call auto-immune or hypersensitivity diseases.

Sometimes the immune system runs wild, and rather than attacking cancer, bacteria, viruses and the like, it attacks the body. A classic example is rheumatoid arthritis. In this condition, the immune system attacks the joints viciously. Sometimes, the system overreacts to otherwise harmless substances. Allergies are the perfect example of this. The immune cells come across pollen and go berserk. They interpret the pollen as a threat and bombard the mucous membranes lining the nose with inflammatory substances. The result, a stuffy nose.

When the immune system overreacts, it can attack any part of the body. The joints, skin and mucous membranes, are the usual targets. Here are some of the conditions that we now know are caused by hyper-immune function, and which the Eclectics treated with *E. angustifolia*.

Chronic skin conditions

The following most remarkable case occurred in my practice:

A gentleman, aged about forty-five years, in apparently good health, was vaccinated, and as the result of supposed impure virus a most unusual train of the symptoms supervened. His vitality began to wane, and he became so weak that he could not sit up. His hair came out, and a skin disease pronounced by experts to be psoriasis, appeared upon his extremities first, and afterward upon his body. In the writer's opinion, the condition had but little resemblance to psoriasis. It seemed more like an acute development of leprosy than any other known condition.

This advanced rapidly, his nails began to fall off, he lost

flesh, and a violent iritis of the left eye developed and ulceration of the cornea in the right set in, and for this difficulty he was referred to Prof. H. M. Martin, President of the Chicago Ophthalmic College.

The condition progressed rapidly towards an apparently fatal termination. At this juncture, Dr. Martin asked the writer to see the case with him. It looked as if there was no possible salvation for the patient, but as a dernier ressort, the writer suggested Echinacea twenty drops every two hours, and the phospho-albusain to be continued. With this treatment, in from four to six weeks, the patient regained his normal weight of more than one hundred and fifty pounds and enjoyed afterward as good health as ever in his life.

Hyperthyroid disease

Dr. Wilkenloh reports the treatment of at least five cases of goitre, three of which had exophthalmic complications, and all were cured, with this remedy alone. The doctor gave the remedy internally in full doses, and injected from five to fifteen minims directly into the thyroid gland, and kept gauze, saturated and applied externally. As no other remedy than this was used, there could be no doubt about its positive influence.

Alopecia

Dr. Hewitt used Echinacea in alopecia. He made a strong solution and combined with it agents that would assist in stimulating the nutritive functions of the hair follicles. He was well satisfied with the result.

These have been a few examples of hyper-immune disease being treated with *E. angustifolia*. Another example we saw earlier was kidney failure following on from scarlet fever. Here too we now recognise an example of an immune system gone wrong. This contradictory use, so common to herbal medicine, is a feature that we still do not understand.

Dosage

As we conclude our survey of the medical legacy bequeathed by the Eclectic movement, let us take one final piece of advice from Dr Ellingwood about the proper use of *E. angustifolia*. This statement is based on fifty years' experience, and we had better take it seriously if we want to equal what these lost pioneers achieved.

> I am convinced that success in certain cases depends upon the fact that the patient must have at times, a sufficiently large quantity of this remedy in order to produce full antitoxic effects on the virulent infections. I would therefore emphasize the statement which I have previously made that it is perfectly safe to give Echinacea in massive doses—from two drams to half an ounce every two or three hours—for a time at least, when the system is overwhelmed with the toxins. This applies to tetanus, anthrax, actinomycosis, pyemia, diphtheria, hydrophobia, and meningitis.

The lesson is: if you want to use *E. angustifolia* in acute disease, use it in massive doses.

The Eclectics used tinctures made from the fresh root, either strong tinctures made from 1 part fresh *E. angustifolia* root and 1 part alcohol (1:1 tinctures), or weaker tinctures in a proportion of 1:5. They also used the fresh root itself. Typical doses are:

Tincture 1:1 =   3 ml per day
Tincture 1:5 = 15 ml per day
Fresh root   =   3 grams per day

Frequency of doses
Acute disease: every half-hour
Chronic disease: every 4 hours

Taking the message forward

You wanted to know more about Echinacea, and I think that you now know more than most people do. This has been a lot of information to take on board, but if you want to use herbal medicines, you need to learn the lessons of their history. Properly used, *Echinacea angustifolia* is a miracle plant, and one of the reasons we spent so much time with the Eclectics is that they were the people who pioneered and refined its use, the only ones who really worked with it in a scientific manner. To know about *E. angustifolia*, you are bound to dip into their work.

Now that you have absorbed this information, I would like to offer a summary of the basic lessons to be taken forward, in the form of some questions and answers. See if you can answer the questions for yourself, before you read the answers!

Eclectic lessons

Q. Which Echinacea species did the Eclectics use?
A. *Echinacea angustifolia.* The Eclectics rejected all other species as inferior.
Q. Which Echinacea species got the clinical trial of all time and passed the Eclectic test?
A. *Echinacea angustifolia.* Though the other species may have merit, the Eclectic Institute did not study them. All we have learned applies to this species exclusively. The Eclectics did not study 'Echinacea', they studied *E. angustifolia*.
Q. What conditions did the Eclectics successfully treat with *Echinacea angustifolia*?
A.
1 Poor immune function:

   a) the inability to fight off infection;
   b) poor healing capacity.

2 Bacterial infection:

   a) all types of bacterial infection;
   b) the symptoms of bacterial infection (i.e. fever, destruction of tissue);

c) prevention of bacterial infection in those exposed to it (i.e. someone exposed to diphtheria or having had surgery).

3 Viral infection:

a) to prevent viral infection taking hold (i.e. rabies after rabid dog bite);
b) to prevent secondary infections following on from viral infections (i.e. pneumonia after influenza).

4 Wounds

a) to prevent wounds from becoming infected;
b) to speed the healing of wounds.

5 Cancer

a) used to an extremely limited extent to treat cancer;
b) Eclectic work suggests *E. angustifolia* needs further investigation in the treatment of cancer.

6 Hyper-immune function

a) skin conditions like eczema, urticaria, allergic dermatitis;
b) auto-immune disease following on from bacterial infections (e.g. streptococcal throat followed by rheumatic joints).

CHAPTER 4

The Modern Age: 1930–1998

With all the excitement surrounding *Echinacea angustifolia* during the Eclectic period, you might expect big things to have happened in the years that followed. Unfortunately, this was not the case. When the Eclectic Institute closed, interest in *E. angustifolia*, and indeed in all of the Echinacea species, disappeared. A silence fell.

The loss of popularity and use was due to more than the extinction of the keenest supporters of this medicinal plant. We saw in chapter 3 that the main Eclectic use of *E. angustifolia* was in the treatment of bacterial infection. In the 1930s, antibiotics came into existence. Suddenly bacterial disease, which had previously confounded the 'regular' physicians and killed most of their patients, could be cured completely with a dose of antibiotic. Suddenly the orthodox physicians had a drug that had a nearly 100 per cent cure rate in bacterial disease. The Eclectics in their heyday had achieved a miraculous 85 per cent cure rate, using *E. angustifolia*. If you had syphilis and could choose between an 85 per cent chance and a 100 per cent chance of being cured, there is no doubt which you would pick. At that time, antibiotics represented a superior drug, and the most effective drug always wins. *E. angustifolia*, no matter how promising, could not compete with antibiotics. They made the plant an obsolete technology.

The years between 1930 and 1960 are best described as the 'Echinacea Dark Ages'. The only people who used *E. angustifolia* were the ageing Eclectic physicians, and with each year that passed there were fewer and fewer of these veterans practising, or indeed living. In this period, the entire focus of medicine became anti-biotics; all of the medicinal plants used previously to deal with bacterial infection got dropped like hot potatoes.

In the 1960s–1970s, the research world turned its attention to cancer. Many medicinal plants were investigated, and those suspected of being 'immune stimulants' were the first to get a review. Science had realised that the immune system was responsible for policing cancer cells. If the immune system could be stimulated, there was the chance that cancer could be controlled. During this period, Echinacea species were studied to a very limited extent. This work was done on a highly academic basis—none of the Echinacea species were being used extensively as a medicine.

In the 1980s, a herbal medicine renaissance started. People became disenchanted with the medical establishment, and started using and studying herbal medicines once again. Early in the renaissance, the Echinacea species reappeared on the scene. Serious drawbacks had emerged with antibiotics, and those who were looking for a herbal alternative found it in this group of plants. Slowly but surely, the various Echinacea species crept into our lives. Books were written, and products introduced. In 1979 Echinacea was a minor product; in 1997 Americans spent $365 million on Echinacea. Echinacea is back, with a vengeance.

Twenty years into this renaissance, it would be nice to say that we have a new stack of Echinacea studies to review, and that great discoveries have been made. Sadly, this is not the case. As we approach the year 2000, we know little more about the plant than was known when the Eclectics finished working with it. Despite Echinacea's current popularity, very little original research has been done on it since those days. Studies in the last twenty years have shown that the various Echinacea species stimulate the immune system. Present-day practitioners will tell you that they help people avoid or recover from infectious disease. This was discovered nearly eighty years ago. In the absence of new information in the modern age, our only verification comes from the work of the Eclectics.

In fact, it could be argued that we have taken a few steps backwards. The Eclectics conducted clinical trials on human beings, in hospitals. The patients took *E. angustifolia* orally; the Eclectics then examined their blood, and monitored their symptoms and conditions. The Eclectics researched the plant's effect on men and women. Today, most of the studies have been done on rabbits, mice and rats. Very few have been done on human beings, and in those that have been done, the human subject has mostly been *injected* with Echinacea extracts. There is a big difference between injecting Echinacea and giving it orally. Despite the advances in technology, scientific studies have not taken us beyond what the Eclectics knew in 1920. In the year when Echinacea had gross sales in America of $365,000,000, one might have expected there to be a bevy of sponsored research studies. This does not appear to have been the case.

One of the problems with the herbal renaissance is that people are dipping into the past in a hit-or-miss manner, with no set methodology and no code of practice. Here is a perfect example. When you talk about the Echinacea species in the modern age, you have to discuss *E. angustifolia* and *E. purpurea*. One of the really odd features of this herbal medicine renaissance is that *E. purpurea* is more commonly used than *E. angustifolia*. This is the case, despite the fact that the Eclectics, the professionals who knew the different species and did more work with them than any other group, dismissed *E. purpurea* as inferior. The prestige of *E. purpurea* is something I find curious. There are two possible answers. The first might be that though *E. angustifolia* fell out of use as a medicine after 1920, *E. purpurea* became a popular garden plant. It was hybridised and developed into a showy addition to any garden border. As the herbal medicine renaissance began, there was lots of *E. purpurea* about—all you had to do was visit the local garden centre.

The second reason why *E. purpurea* is more commonly used today may simply be that it is cheaper. HCR buys the different Echinacea species for our own testing purposes. *E. purpurea* costs £20 pounds a kilo, and *E. angustifolia* costs £50 pounds a kilo. By using the cheaper of the two, the industry can produce a more reasonably priced product.

One of the questions in my mind when I sat down to write this book was how *E. purpurea* became the primary Echinacea used, seeing that the Eclectics so categorically dismissed it. After many hours of interview work, the question remains unanswered. The experts questioned on the matter all scratched their heads and said: 'Don't know.' Sometimes, things in life and society just happen. In this case, not only is *E. purpurea* more widely used, it has been more widely studied in recent times. Many authors lump both species together and refer to them as 'Echinacea' generically. I think this a mistake. When we examine the information that has become available in the modern age, we shall look at these two different plants separately.

A CLOSER LOOK AT THE IMMUNE SYSTEM

Before we look closer at *E. angustifolia* and *E. purpurea*, we need to review the immune system in general terms. Echinacea is an immune stimulant, a means to help the body to help itself. In order to understand the work that has been done in the modern age, we need a basic knowledge of how our immune system works. I have tried to present the concept simply. Earlier, I mentioned that the forces of nature—bacteria, viruses, protozoa and the like—are hungry. They feed on anything organic. If you put a pile of grass clippings on the compost heap, and revisit the heap two weeks later, the forces of nature will have decomposed the clippings to mulch. We have the same forces acting on us. The reason we don't become mulch is that we have an immune system, a comprehensive network of protection that needs to be fuelled and maintained.

Immunity is not automatic. Many of my patients have smoked for decades, yet most of these committed smokers have not developed lung cancer. For some reason their bodies have been able to fight off cancer cells. Likewise, the difference between people becoming HIV-positive or not lies in the power of their immune system. The immune system prevents disease from taking hold. If it is strong, people stay well.

*　　*　　*

For the average person the immune system calls up no definite picture. A structure like the cardiovascular system is more readily understood. It is comprised of the heart, arteries, veins and blood. People can feel their own heartbeat, and see their pulse rise and fall. The cardiovascular system is tangible and therefore easier to perceive and analyse. The immune system, on the other hand, is made up of cells so small that they can only be seen with the aid of a microscope. There is no obvious spot in the body where the immune system dwells. It is essentially silent and invisible, so unobtrusive that for most of human history doctors did not realise it existed.

To grasp the nature of the immune system, it may be helpful to view it as an army. Armies are made up of soldiers; the immune system is made of white blood cells. There are lots of different types of soldiers, experts in different environments—the marines, the navy, the airforce. The immune system has lots of different kinds of white blood cells.

Armies have barracks where the troops live and sleep. The immune system has lymph nodes where the immune cells, the white blood cells, congregate. The immune army, like all armies, is mobile. It directs cells to where trouble can be found. If there is a conflict on the border, the army travels to the border and settles the matter. If you scratch your finger and bacteria enter your body via the broken skin, white blood cells leave the lymph nodes, march down to the finger and zap the intruding bacteria. You can't point to your immune system because on any given day it will be operating in a different location, depending on where it is needed. Today, it might send units to your toe; tomorrow a task force to your ear.

There are two divisions in the Immune Army, the Cellular Mediated Division (CMD) and the Acquired Division (AD). These two armies of the immune system work in harmony to keep the body free of disease. They work together, in the same way that the army might join forces with the navy.

The CMD soldiers are called phagocytes. These cells are front-line soldiers, whose job is to destroy the enemy and ask questions later. The phagocytes are programmed to see body cells as friends and any foreign 'non-body' cell as the enemy. Foreign cells include bacteria and viruses. Cancer cells are cells that have become different from normal cells in the body. Because they are different, they are also seen as enemies. The CMD soldiers are not terribly bright. They spot enemies and kill them. They can differentiate between cells that are supposed to be around and cells that aren't.

The phagocytes have another essential task to fulfil. They function as garbage collectors as well as police. Cells in the body die all the time. The phagocytes collect them and deposit their carcasses in the rubbish bin. These scavenger cells are actually overzealous in their aim of keeping the body tidy. If they notice a cell is in the process of dying, they go ahead and kill it and haul it off to the dump. Normal cells in the body are much like office workers. In the process of doing their job they make a lot of litter. Without the immune cells, the body would quickly become filled with so much litter that work would cease.

Some phagocytes are somewhat like bees. Using a stinger and a pouch filled with venom, they inject the enemy with killing compounds, poisons that cause a fatal meltdown. These are killing machines. Other phagocytes simply swallow their foe, the way a snake consumes a rat—tail and all. This technique is called phagocytosis.

The second division of the Immune Army is the Acquired Division. The AD fields soldiers that are slightly more intelligent. They have a memory. Every enemy is different: some can be killed with a machine-gun, others with a torpedo, and others still require a nuclear bomb. When the soldiers in the AD kill enemies, they remember how they did it. If that particular enemy reappears, they know exactly how to deal with it from prior experience. The nice thing about the AD is that its members can never forget an enemy once encountered. They are called the Acquired Division because they acquire knowledge and put it into use.

The AD group of cells could be seen as the officer contingent. If they come across a problem in the body, they can kill the enemy themselves, but they also call in the CMD for back-up. They direct the CMD cells to a trouble zone and put the foot soldiers into action.

Whereas a conventional army communicates with walkie-talkies and cellular phones, the Immune Army communicates by means known as cellular mediators. When an immune cells comes across a group of enemies, it sends out a message to the rest of the immune system, to alert all soldiers to the problem. Cellular mediators are compounds produced by the immune cell having made contact with trouble. They work a bit like dropping white pebbles in the woods so that a search team can find you. Cellular mediators are little bits of material that attract other immune cells. They might be seen as flares, signals that get the main forces mobilised.

Another part of the Immune Army is the Spy Division. The immune system has agents hidden all over the body that lie in wait for enemies. If they spot an intruder, the spies send out flares to call in the Cellular Mediated Division and the Acquired Division.

The system becomes very interesting, because not only do the immune soldiers communicate with each other through cellular mediators, but citizen cells of the body communicate with the immune soldiers. When a citizen cell becomes infected with a virus, it sends out distress messages to the immune soldiers in the form of proteins known as interferons. The immune cells pick up the message and go to the cell in distress. The interferon message is also picked up by neighbouring citizen cells. It alerts them to lock their doors because there might be other viruses looking to infect them.

This is a highly simplified account of the immune system, but it conveys how the system works in general terms. In fact the Cellular Mediated Division has many different soldiers: phago-cytes, neutrophils, eosinophils and monocytes. The soldiers in the Acquired Division are lymphocytes known as B- and T-cells. The Spy Division is made up of basophils. The most important idea to grasp is that the immune system is a mobile system that roves the body keeping bacteria, viruses, fungi and cancerous cells under control. In the perfect world, the immune system moves to where it is needed, and kills everything that needs to be killed.

With the help of this basic account, the information of *E. angus-tifolia* and *E. purpurea* will make more sense. When we say that

E. angustifolia is an immune system stimulant, we mean that it increases the number of immune soldiers on the beat and strengthens their activity. It works on the body by working with the immune system.

ECHINACEA ANGUSTIFOLIA IN THE MODERN AGE

To examine *E. angustifolia* in the modern age means searching in two different places. First one has to investigate what studies have been done on *E. angustifolia* directly. Researchers have chopped up the plant, made extracts of the bits, and studied what *E. angustifolia* does to animals and to cells in the test-tube. The second approach is to look at what has been learned about the individual constituents found in *E. angustifolia*. Just as we found when trying to understand the Native American use of Echinacea, in order to explore the contemporary research on the plant one spends a lot of time grabbing at straws and piecing together pieces of a jigsaw puzzle. We shall look at these two areas separately, and summarise the new knowledge available to us.

Studies conducted on *E. angustifolia*

Immune activation
In the Ellingwood text in chapter 3, we read that *E. angustifolia* affected both the number of white blood cells and the activity of those cells. To refresh your memory, they determined this by first testing the blood of hospitalised patients, then giving the same patients *E. angustifolia*, and then testing their blood a second time to see if a difference appeared. They found that after treating a patient with *E. angustifolia* they counted more white blood cells, and that these cells were more active. Modern lab work has confirmed the Eclectic finding. Here are some results of recent studies.

- When rabbits were injected with an extract of *E. angustifolia* their white blood cells contained an increased amount of killer substances used to kill bacteria, virus and cancer cells.
- A water-based extract of *E. angustifolia* increased

phagocytosis, the absorption of foreign bodies by the scavenger cells. An alcohol extract was found to more powerfully stimulate phagocytosis than the water extract.

- Alkylamides extracted from *E. angustifolia* increased phagocytosis.
- A tincture of *E. angustifolia* was found to increase the amount of killer substances found in phagocytes.
- An alcohol extract of *E. angustifolia* was shown to increase phagocytosis by 20–30 per cent in mice after oral administration. Large amounts were administered to the mice. Chloroform fractions made of the ethanol extracts were more active than hydropic fractions.
- In mice, alcohol extracts of *E. angustifolia* showed that carbon clearance was increased twofold following oral administration to mice. This proves that phagocytosis is increased in mice, when they are treated with *E. angustifolia*.

Research done in the last twenty years has thus shown that *E. angustifolia* stimulates the white blood cells of rats, mice, and the occasional rabbit. A lot of lab animals lost their white blood cells and more to confirm what the Eclectics established seventy years ago! It's official: *E. angustifolia* is an immune stimulant.

One study in this pile of animal research provides us with some useful information. First, research has shown that the alcoholic extract of *E. angustifolia* is a more powerful immune stimulant than the water-based extract. This means that an alcoholic tincture made of *E. angustifolia* is better than a tea. One study showed that the plant stimulated the immune system when given orally in large quantities. The Eclectics said the same: use *E. angustifolia* in large amounts, and use an alcohol-based tincture.

Bacterial infection
The primary Eclectic use of *E. angustifolia* was to treat bacterial infection. The fact that it has been found to stimulate the white blood cells responsible for hoovering up bacteria explains why the Eclectics found it so effective. Contemporary research has shown

that this anti-bacterial activity is complex, and is due to more than just increased absorption by the white blood cells. In addition, *E. angustifolia* has been shown to have a mild antibiotic effect. This means that the plant contains substances which attack or inhibit bacteria directly. As an example, a complex caffeic acid from *Echinacea angustifolia* roots was found to inhibit *Staphylococcus aureus*. (This is the bacterium responsible for the flesh-melting infections sometimes picked up in hospitals.) In addition, four polyacetylenes in *E. angustifolia* were found to be bacteriostatic. These substances were found to inhibit *E. coli* and *Pseudomonas aeruginos.*

It has to be said that the antibiotic effect of the compounds found in *E. angustifolia* has been described as mild. However, this mild antibiotic effect combined with the immune stimulation also produced by the plant could provide the double whammy we need to fight off a bacterial infection.

Fungal infection
The Eclectics used *E. angustifolia* to treat a small number of fungal infections. Contemporary research validates this use. The same white blood cells responsible for killing bacteria also go after the fungi responsible for certain infections in humans. Beyond this, four polyacetylenes in *E. angustifolia* were found to be fungistatic. As with bacterial infection, when we look at fungal infection and *E. angustifolia* we find another double whammy offer.

Protozoal infection
The Eclectics used *E. angustifolia* to treat a number of protozoal infections, most notably malaria. Malaria continues to be a world-wide killer, and there are good reasons why the modern research community might look at how *E. angustifolia* affected malarial infection. Such is not the case! What has been established is that *in vitro* (in the test-tube) an alcoholic extract of *E. angustifolia* inhibited *Trichomonas vaginalis*, another problematic parasitic infection. This sexually transmitted bug is by no means life-threatening, though it does make being alive a misery.

As with bacterial and fungal infection, the white blood cells are responsible for killing protozoa. We only have one piece of research that suggests *E. angustifolia* inhibits protozoa, though further research may indicate that it inhibits others. *E. angustifolia* may offer the same double protection in protozoal infection as it does in bacterial and fungal infection. As malaria continues to cause the world grief, someone needs to look at this potential use. *E. angustifolia* seeds are cheap, and the plant would happily grow in the areas where malaria is rife and money scarce.

Anti-inflammatory effect

The Eclectics used *E. angustifolia* to reduce all kinds of inflammation, from rattlesnake bite to poison ivy. They found that it was tops when it came to getting the skin to heal. Virtually no research has been done in regard to this well-described use. The sum total of research in this area is that a polysaccharide fraction of *E. angustifolia* displayed anti-inflammatory activity in rats. One study on rats is hardly validation of the Eclectic use, though it is a start.

Anti-cancer effect

As the Eclectic movement was coming to a close, they had begun looking at the role of *E. angustifolia* in cancer. Sadly, they did not get very far before their doors were shut, beyond pointing to its probable utility.

In the modern age there has been virtually no *in vitro* research about the potential anti-cancer activity of *E. angustifolia*, and no *in vivo* (in the person) research either. The only work done to date showed that the essential oil of *E. angustifolia* was found to inhibit Walker carcinosarcoma 256 and P-39 lymphocyte leukaemia. The plant's use in cancer remains uncharted territory, though seeing that the immune system kills off cancer cells, and that *E. angustifolia* stimulates the white blood cells responsible for performing this task, the possibility is not to be dismissed. In this case we are talking about a severely hypothetical use, and one that needs additional research in the lab and in the clinic. The plant is non-toxic, using it would not hurt anyone. It might help, it might not. Only research can tell us.

Conclusion: studies of E. angustifolia *as a whole*
When you look at the modern work on *E. angustifolia* two things become clear. The first is that the Eclectics' opinion of the plant was spot-on, and this opinion has been validated in the modern arena. The second point that comes home is that there is a lot of work that needs to be done. Unexplored areas, such as its activity in cancer, and in infectious diseases like malaria, are crying out for researchers to dig in, and find out if it could make a difference. This plant may offer compounds that can end a lot of suffering worldwide, but work needs to be done to see if this is the case. Generally speaking, where there is smoke there is fire, and clearly *E. angustifolia* is emitting smoky vapours!

Studies conducted on constituents found in *E. angustifolia*
When *E. angustifolia* was analysed in the modern age, the following main groups of compounds were found:

1 caffeic acid derivatives
2 flavonoids
3 essential oil
4 polyacetylenes
5 alkylamides
6 polysaccharides

When modern people look at herbal medicines they are often looking for THE magical constituent that makes it work. This is a mistake, as in fact it is never a single constituent that makes a medicinal plant work. Research has shown, time and time again, that it is different constituents working together that create the ultimate effect of a medicinal plant. *E. angustifolia* has been shown to stimulate the immune system. When you look at the compounds it contains, you find that there is not just one constituent at work, but rather several different groups of compounds, performing combined operations.

Let us delve into these six groups of compounds found in *E. angustifolia* and learn this lesson first-hand.

1 Caffeic acid derivatives

Echinacea angustifolia is rich in substances known as caffeic acid derivatives, that is compounds formed on a base of caffeic acid. Caffeic acid belongs to a family of compounds known as phenols. As various phenols have been found to have antibacterial, antifungal and anti-inflammatory action, this fits nicely into the pattern of uses drawn up by the Eclectics for *E. angustifolia*. Recent work with these substances validates the Eclectic experience. In the 1950s echinacoside was found to have a weak antibiotic activity. Studies show that this substance accumulates in the roots of *E. angustifolia*, though it was recently found in the flowers. Additional studies have shown that echinacoside does not stimulate the immune system, neither increasing the number of white blood cells nor improving their activity. This is an important detail, since many Echinacea product manufacturers are standardising Echinacea products to these echinacosides.

To discuss this point, let me explain standardisation. When manufacturers standardise a product it means they pick one group of compounds found in a plant and then check to make certain their product contains the same amount of that particular substance, no matter what. This may be done at the expense of anything else the plant may contain. If a product was going to be standardised, one would hope it would be to one of the proven active substances. As Echinacea products are used to stimulate the immune system, a product standardised to a group of compounds shown not to stimulate the immune system is counter-productive.

In 1988, verbascoside was found in the leaves of *E. angustifolia*, and it is quite similar to the echinacosides in chemical structure. Research has shown that verbascoside interrupts the usual inflammatory reaction, and thus is a fairly powerful anti-inflammatory substance. If the root contains verbascoside, this may explain why it has the ability to reduce the inflammation experienced with all kinds of venomous bites.

In 1987 cynarin was found in *E. angustifolia*. This substance is unique to the plant, and does not occur in any of the other species of Echinacea. Studies show that cynarin is highly active on the liver, and both increases the activity of the liver and protects it from damage. (This is the same compound that makes the popular milk thistle protect the liver from damage!) Though *E. angustifolia* is not particularly used in liver disease, the presence of this substance makes it a possible candidate to combat liver disease. The activity of cynarin has been shown to be as follows:

cholagogue: increase bile output from the gall bladder
choleretic: increases bile production by the liver
cholesterolytic: breaks down cholesterol
hepatoprotective: protects the liver from damage
hypocholesterolymic: reduces cholesterol levels
hypolipidemic: reduces fat levels in the blood

Though *E. angustifolia* has not been used to treat viral hepatitis in the past, the fact that it contains cynarin strongly suggests it might have a use in such conditions. Milk thistle has worked marvellously in these infectious diseases. The fact that *E. angustifolia* has immune-stimulating as well as liver-protecting properties makes it an ideal medicine for viral hepatitis, which is kept in remission by proper immune function. Let's put this on our 'needs more investigation' list.

In 1984 cichoric acid was found in trace amounts in the root of *E. angustifolia*. Studies have shown that this compound increases the number and activity of the white blood cells and indeed has an antiviral activity.

*   *   *

The caffeic acid derivatives found in *E. angustifolia* have been shown to stimulate the immune system, to be antibacterial, antifungal, antiviral and antiinflammatory. These compounds do a lot of things the Eclectics said *E. angustifolia* did, and then some. There is no coincidence here, and time will probably reveal that the caffeic acid derivatives are essential to the plant's activity.

2 Flavonoids
The Eclectics did not use the leaf of *E. angustifolia*, and contemporary research suggests that this may have been a mistake. Recent

work has revealed that the leaves of the plant are rich in flavonoids, which are highly active. In 1960 the leaves were determined to contain 38 per cent flavonoids.

These substances are interesting because they have been shown to have a wide range of activity in the body. Generally speaking, flavonoids have been shown to reduce capillary fragility and permeability, to mop up free radicals, and to inhibit certain dangerous enzymes. The collective result of these compounds is that they are powerfully anti-inflammatory. The three most interesting flavonoids found in *E. angustifolia* are luteolin, kaempferol and quercetin, whose properties are as follows:

luteolin: antihistaminic, anti-inflammatory, antioxidant, antispasmodic, antitussive, cancer preventer, choleretic, diuretic.

kaempferol: antihistaminic, anti-inflammatory, antioxidant, antispasmodic, antitumour, anti-ulcer, cancer preventer, choleretic, diuretic, HIV inhibitor, retrovirus inhibitor, hypotensive.

quercetin: anti-aggregant, anti-allergenic, anti-anaphylactic shock, antidermatitic, anti-influenza virus, antihepatotoxic, antiherpetic, antihistaminic, antihydrophobic, anti-inflammatory, antileukotrienic, antioxidant, antipermeability, antispasmodic, antiviral, bactericide, cancer preventer, capillariprotectant, HIV inhibitor, retrovirus inhibitor, larvistat, lipoxygenase inhibitor, mast cell stabiliser.

This very preliminary research suggests that the leaves might be beneficial. No clinical research has been done to establish whether they have a medicinal effect; however, it would be illuminating if it was done. The research we have suggests that there is potential here.

This brings up an important lesson. In the modern age we have the opportunity to improve upon the previous uses of medicinal plants. The Eclectics said, discard those leaves. Modern research shows that they might be of use. Modern herbal medicine is about taking information from all sources, synthesising it, and creating a new and improved practice of herbal medicine. When you use historical practices in combination with contemporary research, you end up with a more sophisticated and effective brand of herbal medicine.

3 Essential oil

If you sniff the freshly dried root of *E. angustifolia*, you will notice that it has a distinctive smell. This comes from the essential oils found in the roots. The root contains very little essential oil—in fact less than 1 per cent of its volume—but it seems that not much is required to makes its smell unique.

Essential oils are antibacterial, antifungal and antiviral by nature. The most famous bug-killing essential oil is thymol, found in thyme, and formerly the disinfecting agent used in operating rooms. Bearing in mind that *E. angustifolia* has been used to treat all manner of microbial infections, the fact it contains bug-killing oil should come as no surprise. However, these oils do more than kill microbial invaders. Here is a sampling of the oils that make up the essential oil of *E. angustifolia* and what they have been shown to do. As you will see, we have another ingredient that explains *E. angustifolia*'s reported activity.

palmitic acid: antifibrinolytic.

borneol: pain-killer, anti-inflammatory, liver protector, spasmolytic.

bornylacetate: bactericide, viricide.

germacrene D: pheromonal.

caryophyllene: anti-edemic, anti-inflammatory, spasmolytic.

caryophyllene epoxide: larvicide.

alpha pinene: anti-inflammatory, cancer preventive.

beta pinene: insectifuge.

myrcene: bactericide, insectifuge, spasmolytic.

limonene: anticancer, antilithic, bactericide, insecticide, sedative, viricide.

1,8-pentadecadiene: antitumour.

When you look at the activities of the essential oils found in *E. angustifolia* you see two activities coming up over and over again. First, they are antimicrobial: they kill bacteria, viruses and fungi. Second, they act as anti-inflammatory agents: they reduce inflammation. There is no doubt they are important constituents, and that they contribute to the activities attributed to this medicinal plant.

This raises an important issue, and one that may not be obvious to the newcomer to the world of herbal medicine. Volatile oils are so called because they have a tendency to evaporate, disappear, move on to parts unknown. If you put a drop of olive oil, a fixed oil, on your blouse, and walk around for a day, at the end of the day the oil drop will still be in the fabric. If you put a drop of volatile oil on the same blouse, within an hour it will be gone. As we want to take advantage of the volatile oils found in *E. angustifolia*, we need to make sure that these oils have not evaporated.

The Eclectics said that the best tincture was made out of the fresh root, and that the tincture should then be kept in coloured glass bottles that were well stoppered. This would trap the essential oils in the medicine. Consumers take note: *E. angustifolia* may be made active by delicate oils. Before purchasing a product make certain that these oils have been preserved.

4 Polyacetylenes

Polyacetylenes can be found in many different types of plants and fungi. They are fairly common substances and they have a universal antibiotic activity—that is, they kill microbes on contact. Some botanists argue that plants produce these substances as a means of staying disease-free: that they are part of the plant's natural defence mechanism. Echinacea has been found to contain 2 per cent polyacetylenes, most of them located in the roots.

As we read earlier, four polyacetylene compounds have been isolated from *E. angustifolia* and were shown to be bacteriostatic and fungistatic. These substances mildly inhibited *E. coli*, *Pseudomonas aeruginosa* and *Trichomonas vaginalis*. The antibacterial and antifungal activity of *E. angustifolia* may in part be explained by the presence of the antibiotic principles.

An important fact has surfaced from modern research, namely that the polyacetylenes are destroyed, lost for ever, during long-term storage of the roots, together with their antibacterial action. This means that *E. angustifolia* should be used as fresh as possible. Once again, research confirms the Eclectics in their advice that the tincture be made out of the fresh root, which would still contain these compounds.

5 Alkylamides
E. angustifolia provides the user with a strange mouth experience, and research has shown that this is caused by the alkylamide content of the root of the plant. Just as salt, lemon juice, hot pepper and sugar have their unmistakable signatures, so too does *E. angustifolia* provide the tasters with its own unique effect. Some say that chewing the fresh root results in a tingling sensation, others describe the effect on the tongue as numbing. The sensation is hard to verbalise and is best experienced.

Alkylamides are interesting compounds, specific to the Echinacea species. They have their highest concentration in *E. angustifolia*. These substances have been found to stimulate phagocytosis, the activity of white blood cells, and have been shown to be at least partly responsible for the immune system stimulation experienced when *E. angustifolia* is used.

The research conducted with the alkylamides found in *E. angustifolia* dealt with toxin clearance from the bodies of animals. That is, animals were injected with toxic substances and research showed that when *E. angustifolia* was administered, these substances were more rapidly removed from the system, purged by the action of the white blood cells. Remember that *E. angustifolia*'s longest use was as a treatment for rattlesnake bites. The bite of a poisonous snake injects the body with the venom. The alkylamide compounds, via immune cell stimulation, have been shown to get venomous toxins out of the body before they have the opportunity to cause damage. Consumer message! Make sure the product you use gives you a tingle on the tongue.

6 Polysaccharides

The term 'polysaccharides', literally means many sugars (poly = many, saccharide = sugar). When you enter the world of herbal medicine, you find polysaccharides mentioned a lot, so it is worth while to note what they are and what they do. Sugars are carbohydrates. A good way to think about them is to liken them to grapes. Grapes can either be single or attached to a bunch. When sugars are single they are known as monosaccharides, examples being glucose, fructose and sucrose, sometimes called simple sugars. When these sugars are attached to a bunch of other sugars, the bunch is called a polysaccharide, or multiple sugar. Some people believe that *E. angustifolia* is made medicinally active by its polysaccharides, complex bunches of simple sugars hooked together.

In recent times a number of plants have been shown to contain polysaccharides which stimulate the immune system. These immunity-boosting substances have received much attention from the press, and many people assume that the polysaccharides found in *E. angustifolia* are responsible for its immune-stimulating activity. In fact, of all the substances found in *E. angustifolia*, its polysaccharides have been the least examined. Though it is true that many plants contain polysaccharides that fire up the immune system, and *E. angustifolia* contains polysaccharides, whether or not these sugars make the plant active has yet to be determined.

We know *E. angustifolia* contains an inulin (a stored carbohydrate) which has been shown to stimulate the immune system. The other polysaccharides contained in this plant have not even been named, let alone studied for immune-activating activity. This calls for another consumer warning. As we do not have a clue as to the importance of the sugars contained in this plant, products standardised to these substances may or may not be the way to go.

On the anti-inflammatory side of the equation the sugars found in *E. angustifolia* have some interesting properties. As early as 1971, echinacin B was shown to have a weak antihyaluronidase activity—this term indicates that a substance is both anti-inflammatory and antibacterial. As well, a crude polysaccharide mixture from *E. angustifolia* roots displayed an anti-inflammatory activity in mice when it was applied topically. Whereas we do not know much about the effect of *E. angustifolia*'s polysaccharides on the immune system, we do know that they are anti-inflammatory.

Sugars can be hooked to other chemicals as well as to each other, and we see this in the case of *E. angustifolia*. The plant contains glycoproteins, meaning sugars that are hooked to proteins. Three glycoproteins have been isolated, and this is extremely interesting because certain glycoproteins found in other plants have been shown to stimulate the immune system.

Maitake, shitake and reishi, three immune-system-boosting mushrooms, have all been shown to be made active by the glycoproteins they contain. Research indicates that these glycoproteins trick the immune system into firing up because they remotely resemble substances found on the surface of bacteria. In this case it is a false alarm, but the result is a stimulated immune system. The glycoproteins in *E. angustifolia* have yet to be studied, but it is reasonable to suspect that they operate similarly to those in other plants.

The *E. angustifolia* story is hardly a finished book. As you have probably noticed, there is a lot more to learn. That much is clear when you look at the polysaccharides found in this plant. There is lots of circumstantial evidence that strongly suggests these are important compounds. What we need is some hard cold research that describes their effects. We will put this on our 'wish list' of future developments!

Conclusion: studies of the chemical constituents of E. angustifolia

Much like the studies done on the actual plant, studies of the chemicals found in *E. angustifolia* validate the Native American and Eclectic uses of the plant. Many of the compounds found in it affect the immune system in a positive manner.

There are several important lessons to take away from this section. One lesson is that it is not a single group of compounds that make *E. angustifolia* an immune stimulant, but rather a whole bunch of different ones. These compounds probably work together

103

to yield the total effect the Eclectics and other practitioners have noticed. Another lessons is that more research is needed to measure what these substances do. We are in early days in this regard.

There is a seriously practical lesson here. The herbal medicines industry has become concerned about the need to standardise herbal medicines. They pick up on one group of compounds and standardise to favour that group. In the case of *E. angustifolia*, as we have seen, the jury is still out: experts are still investigating which compounds are the most important. To standardise a product before identifying its most active elements is a mistake. The lesson is as follows. Until further research is conducted, Echinacea products should not be standardised.

Lessons of modern research

These are some key conclusions that we need to take forward from the modern age:

1   Animal research has validated the Eclectic claim that *E. angustifolia* stimulates the production of CMD immune soldiers and increases their activity once they exist.

2   *E. angustifolia* stimulates the immune soldiers responsible for clearing out bacterial infection and contains antibiotic compounds. It is a reasonable plant to use in acute bacterial infection (e.g. tonsillitis) and chronic bacterial infection (e.g. recurring cystitis).

3   *E. angustifolia* stimulates the immune soldiers responsible for clearing out fungal infection and contains antifungal principles. It is reasonable to use it in fungal infections such as *Candida albicans* (thrush) and athlete's foot.

4   *E. angustifolia* stimulates the immune soldiers that fight off protozoal infection. The Eclectics used it to treat malaria. It would be reasonable for those travelling or living in malaria-ridden areas to add it to their antimalarial regime.

5   Though the Eclectics used *E. angustifolia* to treat viral infection, there is little contemporary research in this direction. Research is required, to see if this use is warranted.

6   Evidence suggests that *E. angustifolia* can be used to treat

inflammation. The Eclectics used it in wounds, insect bites and burns. It would be reasonable to apply it topically and use it internally to encourage healing.

7   *E. angustifolia* stimulates the immune soldiers that attack cancer cells. Although no direct research has been conducted on this use in the modern age, the Eclectics suspected it would improve survival rates in cancer patients. This use needs further investigation. As it is non-toxic, it would not harm a cancer patient. Whether it would help is unknown. As I have said earlier, more research is needed.

8   *E. angustifolia* is made active by a whole spectrum of different compounds found in its tissues. Because this is the case, products should not be standardised to one compound at the expense of others until more research is conducted. By favouring a single component, we are likely to diminish others that may be more useful.

9   The volatile oils and polyacetylenes contribute to make *E. angustifolia* an active medicine. These are destroyed in the drying process. Therefore, the best products are those made with the fresh root of the plant, and by methods that conserve these constituents. An alcoholic tincture is probably the best option. Long storage is out when it comes to *E. angustifolia*.

10   Research has shown that the alcoholic extracts of *E. angustifolia* are more powerful immune stimulants than the water extracts. The Eclectics favoured alcoholic extracts, and they are probably the better products.

11   Contemporary research has shown that the leaves of the plant contain powerful anti-inflammatory compounds. If you choose *E. angustifolia* for inflammation, using the whole plant would be advisable.

ECHINACEA PURPUREA

If you take yourself to the health food or herb shop you will find that 80 per cent of the Echinacea products for sale are made out of *E. purpurea*. This is perplexing, as those who pioneered work with the Echinacea species dismissed this species as being 'universally disappointing'. Why is it that *E. purpurea* is the most widely used Echinacea species today? I have previously listed a few reasons. Here may be another that ties in directly to the modern work on *E. purpurea*.

Whereas the Eclectics masterminded the work with *E. angustifolia*, German scientists picked up the work some sixty years later. In 1988, researchers working in Germany did a compare-and-contrast investigation of *E. angustifolia*, *E. purpurea*, and *E. pallida*. In a study conducted on mice, *E. purpurea* was shown to be the most powerful immune-system stimulant of all three species.

The result of this mouse test may explain why the German researchers subsequently focused their work on *E. purpurea*. The question is, does one mouse test invalidate all of the work of the Eclectics? This becomes a debatable issue.

In the same early German work another important fact surfaced, namely that the root of all three species was a far more powerful immune stimulant than the leaf. Contemporary research has shown that when it comes to immune system stimulation, at least in animal studies, the root is the part to be used.

Virtually all of the research work done to date on *E. purpurea* has been done in Germany. This is rather odd, in view of the quantities purchased by consumers in America. Why haven't the American manufacturers sponsored any research? What we know about *E. purpurea* we know through German work, and we owe them a great debt, as many researchers have spent a great deal of time on this plant.

Here you will find a sampling of the results of the studies conducted on *E. purpurea*. There are more available, and the results you see are those that I felt were the most relevant to the consumer using Echinacea products. These studies do give us some food for thought.

Immune system

By and large most of the research conducted on *E. purpurea* has been looking for immune-system-stimulating effects. The Eclectics found in 1920 that *E. angustifolia* activated the immune system. You do not have to wonder why the research community started looking in this direction with *E. purpurea*, whose close relation had been shown to increase both white blood cell numbers and activity a long time ago. Bearing in mind that *E. angustifolia* is an immune stimulant and that both plants are members of the Compositae family, the outcome of research was predictable.

E. purpurea has been found to do two things: first, to stimulate the production of white blood cells; second, to boost their activity once they exist. In a nutshell, *E. purpurea* has been shown to be an immune stimulant. Of course, most of this work has been done on animals. You will have to decide for yourself if it is relevant to humans!

Increase in white blood cell counts

Injection of an *E. purpurea* extract increased the total leucocyte, granulocyte and lymphocyte counts in rabbits.

An *E. purpurea* extract, in the test-tube, caused human blood marrow to differentiate and to produce immune cells.

An *E. purpurea* extract, in the test-tube, caused leukaemic human blood cells to differentiate into mature immune cells.

After an *E. purpurea* polysaccharide fraction was injected into animals, there was an increase in phagocyte count.

Increase in white blood cell activity

An *E. purpurea* extract, in the test-tube, increased the phagocytic index of human granulocytes.

In mice, an ethanol extract of *E. purpurea* root extracts, orally administered, increased phagocytosis. A chloroform extract of the ethanol extract of these extracts was a more powerful activator of phagocytosis than the ethanol extract.

In mice, an aqueous extract of *E. purpurea* showed a stimulation of phagocytosis. The ethanol extract (lipophilic) was found to stimulate phagocytosis more powerfully than the water extract.

In an animal study, the alkylamide fractions of *E. purpurea* increased phagocytosis.

In the test-tube, cichoric acid from *E. purpurea* increased phagocytosis.

In the test-tube, a nitrogen-free polysaccharide extract from *E. purpurea* (EPS) stimulated the mononuclear immune system, stimulated macrophages to behave cytotoxically towards P815 cells, stimulated macrophages to release interleukin 1, and did not stimulate T-cell proliferation.

The injection of an *E. purpurea* extract into twelve healthy human males caused an increase in phagocytosis.

The injection of an *E. purpurea* extract into twelve healthy human males did not cause an increase in activity in NK cells. (NK cells are responsible for clearing up viral infection.)

The oral administration of an alcoholic *E. purpurea* extract into twelve healthy human males increased phagocytosis.

Interpreting studies

If you want to deal with herbal medicines today, you have to be prepared to deal with studies! Salesmen in the health food trade are fond of saying: 'Research has proved this or that.' Most people are impressed by the words: 'A study proved . . .' We need to learn our way around such statements, because they are often misleading. Using the *E. purpurea* studies we have just seen, we can practise being a critic of studies.

On the surface one could say that the research community has established that *E. purpurea* stimulates 'the immune system'. This statement needs to be reviewed with a cautious eye because it is only partially true. A critical consumer will look beneath the surface of studies and delve deeply to see their relevance.

First, the studies conducted on *E. purpurea* have largely been done on animals. Though it is true that rabbits and people have similar immune systems, there is obviously a difference between a rabbit and a person. It would be more accurate to say that in many animal studies *E. purpurea* has been shown to stimulate the immune system, and in a few human studies *E. purpurea* has been shown to be an immune stimulant.

Always ask the question: 'On whom did they test the herbal medicine?'

The next question to ask is: How was the herbal medicine administered in the study? In all but one of the studies listed above, the *E. purpurea* extract was injected into the animals and/or people involved in the study. How many people using *E. purpurea* inject their dose into their veins? Not many. There is a vital difference between swallowing and injecting any substance. Because most of us swallow our *E. purpurea*, only 1 out of 13 studies is relevant to us. The rest miss the mark because the mode of administration is so different from the way we use the herbal medicine.

So when you look at these studies it turns out that only two or three have immediate relevance to human beings. This is often the case with studies 'proving' a herbal medicine works. The next time someone says: 'It's been proved to work', ask on whom—a person or a rabbit?—and how it was administered (the way you would use it?). Become critical. All these studies *suggest* something, which is different from *proving* it. In general terms, they are speculative rather than conclusive.

Bacterial infection

Contemporary writers claim that *E. purpurea* is an active anti-bacterial medicine. Contemporary research reveals why this may be the case. To appreciate our next dose of research, we need a brief account of cell physiology. This will be kept to a minimum, but without some understanding of how the body is strapped together, the research in question won't make sense. (Bear in mind that what follows is a gross over-simplification, designed to help throw light on a particular point.)

In a house made of brick, the bricks are stuck together with mortar. Bodies are made of cells, and the cells are stuck together in a similar way. However, in this case the mortar that holds the cells together is a substance called hyaluronic acid. Hyaluronic acid keeps all of the cells of the body held tightly together, so we don't fall apart at the seams.

When bacteria try to infiltrate the body, they first have to crawl between the cells to gain access. They have to chip away at the mortar. Bacteria are clever little creatures, and a symptom of their cunning is their production of hyaluronidase. This substance is an enzyme that literally melts hyaluronic acid, the very material that holds our cells tightly together. Bacteria use hyaluronidase to pry cells apart, so they can gain access to the body.

This is where *E. purpurea* comes in. An *E. purpurea* extract has been found to inhibit hyaluronidase. This means that *E. purpurea* counteracts bacteria's strategy for gaining access to the body. In effect, it blunts the bacteria's drill. Contemporary practitioners find that the regular use of *E. purpurea* results in chronic bacterial infections disappearing. Research on *E. purpurea* suggests that it does so by disarming the bacterial mode of operation. (By the by, *E. angustifolia* also contains anti-hyaluronidase compounds.)

In addition, like *E. angustifolia*, *E. purpurea* has been shown to have a mild antibiotic effect. This means it contains substances (in the form of caffeic acids and polyacetylenes) which actually attack bacteria directly. Between the indirect inhibition of bacteria, i.e. the inhibition of the hyaluronidase, the direct inhibition of bacteria through antibiotic principles, and the stimulation of the part of the immune system responsible for killing bacteria, it is fairly easy to see why *E. purpurea*, at least hypothetically, would make a difference in bacterial infection in human beings.

The antibacterial activity has not been well tested in humans in controlled experiments, so this use needs further investigation. However, we do have one human study to look at, in which patients suffering from acute viral and bacterial infections received injections of an *E. purpurea* extract. Their blood was drawn and they were found to have an increase in white blood cell count.

Other infectious diseases

Research has shown that *E. purpurea* is active against other micro-creatures that cause infections. The list of microbes inhibited by this plant and its extracts includes fungi and viruses. The illogical part of this story is that the researchers did not bother to test *E. purpurea* against the diseases the Eclectics found effectively treated by *E. angustifolia*. They picked entirely different infections and probably made their work a lot harder than it need have been. Be that as it may, research has revealed that *E. purpurea* does work against infectious disease beyond bacterial infection. Here are a few examples.

Fungus
Four polyacetylenes in *E. purpurea* were found to inhibit troublemaking fungi.

An extract of *E. purpurea* had a total inhibition of *Epidermophyton interdigitale*, a fungus that infects the skin.

Intramuscular injection and topical application of an *E. purpurea* extract decreased the recurrence of vaginal candida in women.

Virus
A lipophilic extract of *E. purpurea* showed an inhibition of the encephalomyocarditis virus and the vesicular stomatitis virus in mouse cells.

Mouse cells treated with *E. purpurea* showed a 50–80 per cent resistance to viral attack against the vesicular stomatitis virus, the influenza virus, and the herpes virus.

In mouse cells cichoric acid extracted from *E. purpurea* was shown to inhibit infection by the vesicular stomatitis virus by 50 per cent.

An aqueous extract of *E. purpurea* was found to have a marked inhibition of the herpes, influenza and polio viruses.

A study conducted in 1992 in Germany showed that patients suffering from flu-like conditions recovered faster when they used a large dose of *E. purpurea* extract (900 mg per day) than those

111

taking a placebo. Those taking less than 900 mg per day recovered at the same rate as those taking the placebo.

A study in 1993 showed that patients recovered more rapidly from flu-like symptoms when either an alcoholic tincture or a pressed juice product was administered.

*   *   *

This work suggests that *E. purpurea* has the ability to inhibit certain fungi and a number of viruses in the test-tube. A very limited amount of work with people suggests that this has some practical application. Patients with flu and candida (thrush) were better when given the extract of *E. purpurea*.

As the immune system fails in the modern age, both viral disease and fungal disease are becoming more of a problem. For this reason, these two uses warrant further review.

Cancer

One of the limited uses of *E. angustifolia* by the Eclectics was as a treatment for cancer. The word 'limited' is chosen here because they did not use the plant widely for this purpose, and only a few references to this use crop up in the texts they left behind. If they barely used that species of Echinacea to treat cancer, we can be certain that they never used *E. purpurea* for this purpose.

In the modern age no research has examined the role of *E. purpurea* in cancer in humans. As there is evidence to suggest that it stimulates the immune system, which combats cancer, you can see why some have recommended its use. However, this action is entirely hypothetical. There is no early history of *E. purpurea* being used to treat cancer, and no contemporary research to suggest that it makes a difference.

It is frightening to discover that some patients are advised to use *E. purpurea* to treat cancer in a systematic way, given the absence of clinical history or research. I have people recently diagnosed with cancer coming into my pharmacy looking for *E. purpurea*. A neighbour or a friend has said it will help. There are

112

many medicinal plants that have been shown to make a difference in cancer, and this is not one of them. Cancer patients would be better off using one of the plants that have both a history of use in cancer and some scientific back-up for this use. (Maitake [*Grifola frondosa*] is an example.)

Healing wounds

In trawling through the Eclectic work, we saw listing after listing of *E. angustifolia* being used to heal wounds and ulcers. Though they never used *E. purpurea* for this purpose, research has revealed that this plant might be of use, due to the chemicals found in it. This activity brings us back to *E. purpurea*'s ability to inhibit hyaluronidase, the enzyme produced by invading bacteria to melt cells.

Bacteria are not the exclusive producers of this destructive enzyme. The body itself produces hyaluronidase. You may wonder why it would produce a substance that can damage its own cells. The answer lies in the daily behaviour of the body, which is constantly building and demolishing cells. Like old buildings in a city centre, sometimes old cells need to be removed and replaced with new cells. The body produces hyaluronidase to accomplish this task.

Sometimes the body runs riot, and produces too much hyaluronidase. The result can be chronic ulcers and slow-healing wounds. The body literally melts itself. It is possible that topically applying Echinacea would inhibit the surplus hyaluronidase, and that with this destructive enzyme deactivated, healing would occur. There have been several studies where an extract of *E. purpurea* inhibited the body's output of hyaluronidase. As an example, two polysaccharide fractions from *E. purpurea* were found to produce this effect.

In one experiment, a polysaccharide fraction of *E. purpurea* promoted wound healing in animals.

The effect of expressed juice extract of *E. purpurea* was studied in wounds. Hyaluronidase from body cells and that produced by streptococcal bacteria was inhibited by this *E. purpurea* extract.

It had a direct anti-hyaluronidase activity, and was found to be as effective as cortisone as an anti-inflammatory.

In animals, a polysaccharide fraction from *E. purpurea* was shown to promote wound healing due to its anti-hyaluronidase activity.

In wound-healing experiments with animals, there was a reduction in oedema and subcutaneous haemorrhage when an extract of *E. purpurea* was topically applied.

In a study conducted in 1978, 4,500 patients with chronic skin complaints were given an ointment made of *E. purpurea*. Of these, 85 per cent had a positive reaction.

In 1979 another study involving 109 patients confirmed that the plant had healing properties in skin complaints.

Allergic inflammation

There are a number of situations in which the body actually damages itself. This happens in allergic reactions, which are triggered when the immune cells come across something they don't like, and shoot their acid load at the intruder. Only in this case, rather than being a cancer cell, bacterium or virus, the target is harmless: possibly washing up liquid, or a grain of pollen, sitting on the skin or the lining of the nose.

A case of poison ivy might be described as the ultimate allergic reaction. Poison ivy contains compounds which really irritate the immune system. The white blood cells converge on the tissue tainted with the poison ivy oils and spray them with their battery acid. In an average allergic reaction they do this to a limited extent and all you end up with is a small amount of inflammation. In the case of poison ivy the white blood cells do not let up. They keep spraying their acid until the tissue starts to melt. A patch of skin exposed to the poison ivy oils rapidly deteriorates into a mass of ulcers and sores. It is not the poison ivy that inflicts so much damage, but rather the immune system's response to the presence of these oils.

Remember that the Eclectics used *E. angustifolia* to treat poison ivy eruptions. There has not been any modern research looking

114

into the anti-inflammatory activity of *E. angustifolia*, but there has been some for its kissing cousin, *E. purpurea*. Research has revealed that compounds found in *E. purpurea* alleviate this reactionary or inflammatory process.

Here are some further examples of the anti-inflammatory properties of *E. purpurea* or its individual compounds:

- A complex polysaccharide was found to have a cortisone-like activity.
- An alkylamide was shown to be anti-inflammatory.
- Whole extract of *E. purpurea* exhibited an anti-inflammatory effect, equal to cortisone.

You will notice two comparisons to cortisone. Cortisone is used in all anti-inflammatory conditions: asthma, eczema, psoriasis and rheumatoid arthritis are notable examples. It puts the immune soldiers soundly to sleep and when they sleep they stop their mistaken attack. Cortisone is a powerful and effective immune depressant. To learn that *E. purpurea* has been shown to be equally effective is impressive, all the more so because while cortisone unfortunately has a lot of unpleasant side-effects, *E. purpurea* does not. The animal studies suggest that *E. purpurea* needs to be well studied, as it may offer an alternative to cortisone.

Lessons on *Echinacea purpurea*, learned in the modern age

1   *E. purpurea* has been shown to be an immune stimulant in animals. In extremely limited studies it has been shown to stimulate the human immune system.

2   Animal research has shown *E. purpurea* may be a potential antibacterial, antifungal drug, owing to its immune-stimulant activity and the antibiotic principles it contains.

3   Research indicates that *E. purpurea* might be a valuable antiviral medicine. At present, little human work has been carried out, but evidence suggests that it should be.

4   There is no hard evidence that *E. purpurea* is an effective treatment in cancer. It might work or it might not. More research is needed to explore this possibility.

5   Research indicates that *E. purpurea* might be an effective wound-healing agent in humans.

6   Research indicates that *E. purpurea* might be helpful in allergic reactions in humans.

7   In one human study, researchers found that *E. purpurea* was effective in viral disease when used in large amounts.

8   One study showed that the root of *E. purpurea* was the most medicinal part of the plant.

*   *   *

Echinacea pallida.   The third Echinacea species you are likely to encounter at the health food shop, *E. pallida*, is truly the forgotten species. The Eclectics did not mention it at all. The modern research community has spent about the same amount of time on this species as did their predecessors. All said and done, a meagre three studies talk about this plant, and always in relation to its more notable cousins.

The complete silence on *E. pallida* means that we simply do not know much about it. It may be a sleeper, a plant that research shows is the best of all three. However, in the meantime there is no historical or contemporary work to suggest we should use it. If you come across a product that contains it, bear in mind that it is a dark horse, and until someone does some work on it, we do not know how effective it is.

CONCLUDING THE MODERN AGE

We have come to the close of our modern account. This has been a lot of information to look at and digest. Herbal medicine is a fascinating study, because it involves so many different disciplines. You have to learn about medicine, physiology, chemistry and botany! The care and maintenance of the human body is a never-ending story, which calls for our closest attention.

Modern people want things made simple and easy, but life

refuses to be simple. If you want to understand herbal medicine and be able to use it effectively, you have to juggle the facts and disciplines. We are in the process of rediscovering the subject, and this requires studying, learning and thinking. The ultimate objective of looking at all this information has been to get to the bottom of our original list of questions:

1 Which species of Echinacea should be used?
2 What conditions should it be used for?
3 How should we use it?

I shall now present the conclusions I have drawn, based on the information available. You may agree with me, or you may disagree. Either way, you will have digested the information and formed your own opinion.

Which Echinacea species should be used?

When we started out, we were talking about three different species of Echinacea. We shall now narrow it down to one.

E. pallida is easy to discard; there is so little information about it that we can hardly review it. No one has really studied it, so it is impossible to say. Before you decide on a product, you need some basis for use. This species has neither history nor laboratory research behind it.

When we approach *E. angustifolia* and *E. purpurea*, things become more controversial. This contest is not as clear-cut. *E. angustifolia* was the preferred species of the Eclectics. The Germans prefer *E. purpurea* and have done most of their research on this species. This is a difficult one.

My own conclusion is that *E. angustifolia* is the species to be selected and used. Here are my reasons for this. First, this species is the one with the longest history of use and the most detailed record of real human research. The Native Americans used it. The Eclectics studied it for eighty continuous years, and they really studied it from top to bottom. Contemporary research validates this earlier work. The Eclectics used it in the hospital setting for many years, and kept track of the results.

E. purpurea, on the other hand, has been looked at in the labora-

117

tory and has some human research behind it. It may have accumulated ten studies on human beings, looking at its efficacy in disease and in health, but that amount of work pales in comparison to how much time the Eclectics spent on the other species. These studies indicate that *E. purpurea* is worth using. They do not indicate that it is the best species to use.

The Eclectics were the only people who really looked at the two plants from a clinical perspective over a long period of time. They concluded, after using both, that *E. angustifolia* was the superior plant. No subsequent work has proved otherwise.

The handful of studies that show that *E. purpurea* is a more powerful immune stimulant dealt with animals. In my book animals studies take second place to human studies. There are those who will argue this point, but, as far as I'm concerned, a rabbit injected with *E. purpurea* is less relevant than a person fed with *E. angustifolia*.

Clearly more work needs to be done to examine these two species in human beings. Until then, we shall have to go with the biggest pile of clinical research available, and for the time being, that pile belongs to *E. angustifolia*.

Now, for the consumer, this has some serious consequences. At present, *E. angustifolia* costs double what the other species do. As ever, you get what you pay for. Whether you take the plunge and use the more expensive Echinacea will be a personal decision. All I can say is, I use *E. angustifolia* and would recommend that others do the same. In my clinical practice I have found that it wins out over *E. purpurea*.

What conditions should be treated with *E. angustifolia*?
The common thread running throughout the Eclectic use of *E. angustifolia* and the findings of contemporary research is immune system stimulation. Bacterial, viral and fungal infection, as well as wounds, all improve when the immune system gets a boost. The limited amount of contemporary research available confirms that the improvement the Eclectics noticed was down to this activity. *E. angustifolia* is an immune stimulant.

The immune system stands between us and disease, by fighting of bacterial, viral and fungal invaders and healing wounds and

118

sores. As *E. angustifolia* has been established as an immune stimulant, it clearly has a place in the treatment of all of the previously mentioned conditions. As the immune system does so much, the uses for this plant are endless, and its applications unlimited. Here is a list of uses that seem reasonable, based on the available information. This is only my list; use your imagination and new-found knowledge to expand it.

Established uses

1 *Bacterial infection*

- Chronic–cystitis, sinusitis, tonsillitis, etc.
- Acute–cystitis, tonsillitis, pneumonia, etc.

2 *Preventing bacterial infection*

- use prior to a trip to a disease-ridden country, and as a travel aid
- use before surgery
- use before the cough and cold season
- use before visiting a sick person

3 Healing wounds

- apply to a cut and use internally to speed healing
- use on varicose ulcers, internally and externally
- use on surgical wounds, internally and externally, to speed healing and prevent infection

Speculative uses

This list of possible uses is suggested by the information on hand, and by the known general properties of the plant, but in the absence of extended clinical trials, the jury is still out. *E. angustifolia* would not worsen the condition, because it is non-toxic. The extent to which it will help is unknown.

1 *Cancer*

- as an added tool in a cancer-fighting programme
- as a tool to prevent a recurrence of a cancer
- as a tool for those predisposed to cancer

2 *Auto-immune disease*

- rheumatoid arthritis
- lupus
- Reiters' syndrome
- ankylosing spondylitis
- psoriasis

3 *Hyper-immune diseases*

- eczema
- asthma
- hay fever
- allergies

4 *Viral disease*

- to keep viral disease in remission (hepatitis B and C, ME, herpes, HIV)
- to prevent follow-on disease from an acute viral infection (e.g. preventing influenza from becoming pneumonia, etc.)
- to prevent kicking up viral disease (use it during flu season)

How should *E. angustifolia* be used?
Here are some guidelines to using this marvellous medicinal plant.

- The best approach would be to use the fresh root. It should be cleaned and chewed. This is not practical for 95 per cent of the world population, so we turn to Plan B.
- The second best way to use *E. angustifolia* is in the form of a tincture, made of the fresh root. Tinctures are made with alcohol, which helps to preserve the constituents.

How much should be used?
The Eclectic tradition, and contemporary research, indicate that *E. angustifolia* needs to be used in large amounts, especially in acute disease. In non-acute disease, smaller doses should be used. Here is a guideline:

fresh root	3 g per day
dried root	1.5 g per day
tincture 1:1	3 ml per day
tincture 1:5	15 ml per day

This guideline is meant to assist you whilst wading through the health food shops, and very much represents the ideal. Now you know how you should use *E. angustifolia* in the best case scenario. If you only have access to dried *E. angustifolia* root, use it.

It is important for the consumer to demand the best—even if he or she does not get it.

CHAPTER 5

Echinacea: A Classic Tonic Plant

In this book, we started by considering Echinacea as a whole, and looked at all the species. Then we surveyed the history of their medicinal uses. As the pages passed, we became more and more focused, to the point where we were able to specify a species, a series of uses, and a manner of use. Now the time has come to widen the topic again, and to set our understanding of Echinacea in the wider context of preventive medicine. More and more people in the medical world have come to realise that it is better to prevent diseases in the first place, by strengthening the body's own resources, than to wait till they invade, and then resort to drastic measures that may have serious drawbacks for the user.

Preventive medicine is very much coming into its own as we approach the year 2000. Most people would rather stay well than deal with an illness once it exists. This is driving people to the gym, the produce section of the supermarket, and to the health food shop, where consumers are buying boatloads of herbal medicines in the hope of staying well.

When I think about the Echinacea species, I think of what a perfect addition they are to a 'staying well regime'. Yes, they can be used to treat a host of diseases, but they are probably better used to prevent disease in the first instance.

Echinacea angustifolia is a classic tonic plant. What does this mean? Here I would like to explore an approach to health that will augment whichever preventive regime you have under way, or have been planning. Let's talk tonic plants, and how they fit into the picture.

For most of us enthusiasts for herbal medicine, the word 'tonic' is the vaguest of labels. Most commonly, we find it associated with another word, gin, as in gin and tonic. In fact, the sparkling part of that popular cocktail comes straight from the days when tonics were a way of life. Tonic water contains quinine, an extract of *Cinchona rubra*, a classic tonic plant.

As the white colonials snatched up different parts of the globe, they met more opposition than the rightful human owners of the real estate they snatched. Strange types of microbes lived in these foreign lands, and many colonials did not survive the encounter. One of the biggest killers was malaria, the infectious disease spread by mosquitoes. When the Spanish conquistadors made their way into what would become known as Latin America, they were hit by killer malaria. The Native American healers taught the Spanish doctors that if those at risk drank a tea brewed from the bark of *Cinchona rubra*, malaria would not take hold. The Spaniards took this helpful tip on board. They shared the information and the bark with the other European cultures who were also encountering malaria in their expansionist activities.

In time, the colonials discovered that quinine-tinged water prevented a host of diseases found in the tropics. They called this 'tonic water'. When the British made their way to India their biggest foe was infectious disease. Drinking tonic water became a part of the daily routine there. The British like their drink, and have never been known for their love of soft drinks. To right the situation, they combined tonic water with another long-used European health fortifier, gin, to create a powerful disease-preventing beverage. The gin and tonic first came about as a means of staying alive. Today it is just a cocktail; in those days it was an insurance policy against dying of disease in foreign lands.

In the nineteenth century there was a class of medicinal plants, tonics, of which quinine was one, that were used to keep the body strong and able to resist disease. The tonic of 'gin and tonic' fame was only one of many that were commonly used to prevent disease. The fields, woods and mountains were scoured for plants that could be used in mankind's bid to stay well.

At that time, the idea of taking a herbal medicine to maintain health was a well accepted practice. In the *Century Dictionary*, published in 1889, we find tonics defined as: 'medicines increasing the strength and tone of the animal system; obviating the effects of weakness or debility, and restoring healthy function; hence, bracing and invigorating to the mental or moral nature.'

Eclectic medical textbooks from that same period state that tonics, in some inexplicable manner, coax the body towards health and away from illness. In Dr J. M. Scudder's medical textbook, written in 1883, we find a typical reference to tonic plants: 'We may say in reference to this class of agents, that their use is indicated whenever the system is depressed below its normal level. They act directly in support of the vital force, they therefore assist nature in the removal of disease.'

Was Dr Scudder the only Eclectic physician working with tonic medicines in the last century? The answer is no. A careful review of other physicians' views on tonics might help bring the concept into closer focus:

'Medicines that increase the strength or tone of the animal system.'—Dr Howard Horton, MD, 1879.

'Remedies intended to strengthen the system.'—Dr A. W. Chase, MD, 1884.

'Tonics are remedies which moderately exalt the energies of all parts of the body, without causing any deviation of healthy function. While stimulants are transient in their influence, tonics are comparatively permanent.'—Dr R. V. Peirce, MD, 1895.

'A medicine that gradually restores healthy action, that gives strength.'—Dr W. J. Truitt, MD, 1914.

The doctors of that day said that tonics, as a group of medicines, distinguished themselves from other groups of medicines (e.g. laxatives, diuretics, antiseptics, etc.) in their ability to generally strengthen the body. The strong body was less subject to disease. These doctors were not talking theory, they were speaking about what they observed in their clinical practice of medicine. Patients who took tonics were healthier. They simply did not fall ill as often as those patients who did not take tonics.

If you read further into the Eclectic physicians' texts, you notice that this strengthening activity was of great interest to them. They did not understand how tonics worked, and wanted to unearth the how and why. In many ways they were confounded by tonics, though this did not stop them from using them.

In Dr Scudder's definition of tonic we see him use the words 'vital force'. It is a phrase that will appear again and again in connection with the tonic plants of the nineteenth century. The physicians of the day felt that the 'vital force' was like a flame burning within a person. When the flame burned bright, disease was kept out. When it sank low, disease crept into the physical frame. When it went out, life ended. Their theory was that if the flame could be turned up, disease could not get a hold on the body. Tonics were thought to act like petrol poured onto the flame of life. They turned up the brilliance of the 'vital force', which in turn made the body impervious to disease.

We tend to think that the 'new age' and its esoteric thinking is something new. When one explores the world of tonic plants, one finds this is not the case. The Eclectic tonic doctors got pretty abstract in their attempts to explain tonics. The 'flame' theory of the 'vital force' is the most straightforward. To others it resembled a vibration. When the spirit vibrated, one lived; when it lost its resonance, one died. These physicians felt that disease was caused by low vibration. In their view, tonic plants increased the vibration of the spirit, which in turn resulted in vigorous health.

The doctors were seeking a way to rationalise what they saw in their day-to-day practice, namely that patients given tonic plants were stronger, fitter, and less prone to illness. The idea of tonics stimulating the vital force or balancing vibrations explained what they saw in clinical practice and put them more at ease with their use. The truth was that they did not understand the clinical phenomena before them.

To sum up the position, tonics were a group of drugs that doctors used to stimulate strong health in their patients. If you were about to embark upon a trip into a disease-filled locale, they were pre-scribed to make certain you made the return trip. If there was disease in the house, those not yet afflicted were prescribed tonics so that they might not come down with the plague du jour. The doctors working with tonics did not understand them, but all acknowledged that they worked and all took advantage of their inexplicable vitality-inducing power.

In the tonic days, there was a second class of drugs well known to Eclectic physicians. These were called alteratives, and the name is descriptive: alteratives were used to alter the usual course of a disease. Much as with tonics, the doctors using these medicinal agents did not have a clue how they worked. Their clinical practice showed that the usual outcome of a disease was altered when alteratives were administered, and that was good enough for them. We have heard mention of alteratives previously, but we need to go into greater depth.

Here are a few examples. If a person contracted syphilis, he or she normally died a slow and tortured death. When an alterative was used, the syphilis patient lived a reasonably long and healthy life. When a person developed rheumatoid arthritis, the joints were slowly but surely destroyed. When an alterative was used, the expected joint erosion did not occur. Once a child developed eczema, the prognosis was that he or she would suffer from problematic skin throughout life. When alteratives were used, the skin cleared and any remnants of the disease faded away. Alteratives changed the usual course of affairs in a chronic disease.

A quick glance at some medical texts from the nineteenth century may shed additional light on a rather elusive concept. It seems an odd group of medicines to the modern person, but in those days alteratives were seen as standard treatments. Here are some definitions.

'A remedy which gradually restores healthy action to the body.'— A. W. Chase, MD, 1884.

'Causing alteration: having the power or tendency to alter, especially in medicine, having the power to restore the healthy functioning of the body. One of a group of medicines the physiological action of which is somewhat obscure, but which seems to modify the processes of growth and repair of various tissues.'—*The Century Dictionary*, 1889.

'Alteratives are a class of medicines which in some inexplicable manner, gradually change certain morbid actions of the system, and establish a healthy condition instead. They stimulate the vital processes to renewed activity, and arouse the excretory organs to remove matter which ought to be eliminated. They facilitate the action of the secretory glands, tone them up, and give a new impulse to their operations, so that they can more expeditiously rid the system of worn-out and effete materials. In this way they alter, correct, and purify the fluids, tone up the organs, and re-establish their healthy functions.'—Dr R. V. Peirce, MD, 1895.

The critics of alteratives will be quick to label them 'old wives' tales'. One of the chief reasons for this judgement is that the same alterative would have been used to treat so many different diseases. If you look at the old medical books it is not unusual to read that an alterative could be used to treat tuberculosis, cancer, asthma, snakebite, poisoning and gangrene. Rather than being used to treat a specific disease, alteratives were multipurpose. The general nature of alteratives poses a problem for the modern thinker, and sadly, rather than thinking creatively, this group of drugs is dismissed out of hand.

Much as with tonics, the Eclectic doctors said that alteratives worked in an inexplicable manner. They hypothesised that alteratives also stimulated 'life force' and drove disease out of the body by doing so. Disease could not cling to the body when alteratives were added to the equation. Beyond this, they did not understand them. Our inclination today is to discount what we do not understand. These doctors were more practical. Alteratives worked. If they would do some good, the doctors used them.

Tonic or alterative? Those who read old medical books know that there was a lot of cross-over with these curious agents, and in fact the line between a tonic and an alterative is pretty vague. *E. angustifolia* will be called a tonic in one book, and an alterative in the next. What matters is that both tonics and alteratives were seen as agents that improved health and vitality. You could say that tonics stimulated health so that disease could not take hold, and that alteratives helped the body shake off disease once it was entrenched.

In all cases, the huge amount of time and energy these physicians dedicated to finding, studying and writing about tonic and alterative plants says something. Clinicians know when a medicine works and when it does not. This is as true today as it was then. Some called this inexplicable group of medicines tonics and others alteratives. For the sake of ease, from here on these plants will be referred to as tonics.

History of tonic plants 1900–2000

Despite their popularity, and the attention they received in the nineteenth century, people stopped using tonic and alterative plants in the early years of the twentieth. Why shut the door on these plants? Because in the twentieth century something dramatic happened. Medical science advanced so far that it could cure disease. For example, antibiotics were discovered. Tonsillitis, formerly a killer, became a minor aggravation. Surgery was perfected. Heart disease could be fixed with the knife. The focus of the medical community and general public changed from prevention to cure. Tonics and alteratives, like the horse and buggy, were tossed aside for what seemed a simpler option.

Throughout the twentieth century, medical science made one mind-boggling advance after another. The more medical science was able to cure disease, the more people turned away from prevention and tonic plants. Why bother boiling up a pile of Echinacea to keep the kids from picking up tonsillitis, when you could run to the doctor and get a bottle of antibiotics? Tonic plants were abandoned for easier, simpler options provided by the medical community.

As we approach the twenty-first century, tonics are being picked out of the compost heap, dusted off and used. If they went out of favour in 1900, why they are back in favour in 2000? First and foremost, people are turning their attention to prevention, and disease-preventing herbal medicines, for the same reasons they used them in the last century. They have no choice. Staying well is once again a priority; falling ill is not an option for many.

Moreover, the antibiotics that displaced the older methods have stopped working in many cases.

Behind the revival

There are many reasons why tonics are of interest once again, and the common denominator is that people want to stay well and avoid disease if they can. History has repeated itself. Prevention went out at the end of the nineteenth century and is back in at the end of the twentieth. There is no doubt that these plants are back in style. The sales figures for Echinacea alone reveal a major shift.

Often people ask the question, do tonics work? This is the big question, and one that HCR is looking into day and night. Members of the HCR team will tell you that when patients use tonic plants, they feel, look and *are* much healthier. In fact, we ourselves, despite a gruelling workload, don't seem to get sick when taking tonics. Dr Denise Turner, the biochemist in the group, recently remarked: 'Under normal circumstances, the pace we keep would result in me coming down with a lot of colds. Using tonics, I have avoided getting a cold for a long time. Tonics work.'

Our extensive work with tonic plants such as Echinacea indicates that they do what the doctors of the last century said they did. They improve health, prevent disease, and cure existing disease. Scores of patients calling into our London clinic have experienced improvement in their health by using tonics. From a clinical perspective, there is no doubt that tonics work. The issue remains, how do they work?

As you know, doctors in the nineteenth century felt that the improved health enjoyed by those taking tonic plants derived from an increase in 'life force'. Whether these plants' ability to stimulate strong health is due to increased life force is something 'The Herbalists' sit around the lunch table and debate. Until the nature of life is better understood we are unlikely to verify the hypothesis proposed by the long-dead doctors.

When life force can be monitored, we may be able to see what tonic plants do to it. In the meantime we have to work within the limitations of the present scientific world. Research has revealed that these plants do improve health on many different levels and often have a wide and varied activity. Take *E. angustifolia* as an example. This plant and the constituents found in it have been shown to:

1) Stimulate the immune system.
2) Inhibit bacteria, fungus and virus.
3) Increase the liver's cleansing of the blood and its excretion of waste.
4) Protect the all-important liver from damage.
5) Reduce cholesterol levels.
6) Act as an antioxidant.
7) Contain compounds which may prove to be anti-cancer.
8) Stimulate the kidneys to filter out waste more effectively.

With all these activities going on at the same time, it is not hard to see how *E. angustifolia* would improve health. The fact that it improves the excretion of waste would alone engender better health. Despite these findings, we at HCR feel there is a lot more to *E. angustifolia* than research has yet revealed, and that more research is required to fully understand what we see in our clinical practice—namely, improved vitality.

Tonics have specific talents
If you look into the medical books from the nineteenth century you will find 200 different tonic plants listed there. That is a lot of plants. The work done by 'The Herbalists' up to this point has revealed there is a common thread running between all tonic plants, namely that as a consequence of different physiological actions they generally improve health. Beyond this, they have individual actions. Much like people, tonics have attributes that are specific and unique.

Particular tonic plants will specifically prevent damage to a specific system and improve its functioning. Some tonic plants boost the functioning of the respiratory tract and others the digestive system. These targeting activities are not a matter of debate, they are proven facts. A look at the following long-used tonic plants illustrates this point.

Hawthorn: heart disease preventer.   High blood pressure contributes to the development of heart disease. Hawthorn has been shown to reduce blood pressure. Free radicals, naturally-occurring substances produced by life processes, damage the blood vessels serving the heart and lead to atherosclerosis. Hawthorn contains the antioxidant hyperin, which mops up free radicals before they have a chance to damage the blood vessels. Heart disease develops as a result of plaque formation on the interior of the blood vessels, which eventually blocks blood-flow. When the blood can't make it to the heart, heart attacks occur. Rutin, a compound found in hawthorn, reduces plaque formation.

Milk thistle: liver disease preventer.   Research in the lab has shown that a group of chemicals, collectively known as silybin, have a strong ability to protect the liver cells from chemical damage. These flavolignans' ability to accomplish this been confirmed in the lab and in clinical trials. One of the constituents of milk thistle, silymarin, has been shown to be both antiviral and anti-cirrhotic. This antiviral activity explains milk thistle's ability to prevent damage to the liver when people suffer from viral hepatitis.

Liquorice: respiratory disease preventer   Liquorice contains a wild cocktail of compounds that make the respiratory tract function better. Glycyrrhetic acid, glycyrrhizic acid, and glycyrrhizin are the most notable constituents. These compounds have been shown to be anti-inflammatory, antiviral, antibacterial, anti-allergic, and anti-asthmatic. Liquorice has been shown to be antiviral and to stimulate the part of the immune system responsible for attacking viruses. (Let us not forget that coughs, colds, and influenza are caused by viruses!)

Immune tonics
As you can see, there is a tonic for every system of the human body, and this includes the immune system. Whereas the allopathic medical world has little to offer the person looking for immune reinforcement, the world of herbal medicine is rich in plants—used for centuries as tonics—which are being proved to stimulate

the immune system to renewed activity. The list includes Echinacea, Maitake, Astragalus, Pot Marigold, and Achillea. Many of the top-selling herbal medicines today are in fact immune-system tonics. This brings us to *Echinacea angustifolia*. *E. angustifolia* is not the only immune tonic available, and in fact it is only one of many immune tonics available. However, it is one of the best.

In the classic case of Echinacea, we find a situation seen over and over again in the history of the different immune tonics. *E. angustifolia* was first used by the Native Americans to treat snakebite. They found that when a snakebitten person used *E. angustifolia* the venom did not have the usual life-threatening effect. Those bitten did not die.

When the colonials made their way to America they too fell victim to the bites of rattlesnakes and copperheads. The Native Americans introduced them to *E. angustifolia*. More than one pioneer lived to tell the story of having been bitten by a rattler, and using *E. angustifolia* to counter the effects of the venom. The colonials extended the practice, and found the plant effective in all venomous bites and stings, including bees, spiders and wasps.

In the late nineteenth century, doctors felt that bacteria killed a person when they moved into the body and started producing venom which in turn made a person fall ill. Having used *E. angustifolia* successfully to treat snake venom poisoning, it seemed logical to give it a try in bacterial venom poisoning. It worked, and it became the chief treatment for infectious disease amongst certain physicians.

By the end of the nineteenth century *E. angustifolia* was used to treat snakebite, spider bite, tonsillitis, bronchitis, rabies, cholera, diphtheria, tuberculosis, syphilis, gangrene, herpes, chicken pox, mumps, and even cancer. At that time doctors felt that cancer was caused by bad blood, and that it could be cured by using blood-cleansers. *E. angustifolia* had the ability to get venom out of the blood, and as such it was considered a blood-purifier. The doctors used *E. angustifolia* in cancer to a limited extent.

To the modern scientific type, the idea that a plant could treat all of these diseases seems crazy. That is until you go beyond the obvious and think creatively. All of the aforementioned conditions are improved when the immune system is stimulated. The immune cells clean out the venom injected into the body in a snakebite, they kill the bacteria causing tonsillitis, and they destroy cancerous cells. It may seem unlikely that a medicinal plant could treat so many conditions, that is until you realise that the plant is stimulating the immune cells, whose whole purpose is to deal with these conditions.

Contemporary research has shown that *E. angustifolia* does indeed stimulate the immune system. Its constituents increase the production of white blood cells and boost their activity. Lab work has shown that the doctors of the nineteenth century were well advised to use *E. angustifolia* in that long list of diseases. An active immune system would improve all of them.

This has been the story with traditional tonics over and over again. In studies of plants used to treat a host of diseases, modern research has traced the scope of their activity to immune stimulation. It would be appropriate to say that *E. angustifolia* is the most famous and widely used immune tonic, but it is by no means unique in its action.

Problems confronting the immune system

Poor immune function is the scourge of the modern age. The immune army is not making the rounds as it was meant to do. An endless stream of patients suffering from poor immunity floods into the offices of health care practitioners. People suffering from chronic tonsillitis, chronic urinary tract infections, AIDS, cancer, ME and hepatitis are a constant source of aggravation and angst for those whose business is keeping people well. The immune system is failing, and there are few working in medicine who would argue that this is not the case.

'The Herbalists' feel the problem is rather complicated. First, the human immune system is being depressed by the lives we lead. The system is worn out when the day is over. I think it would be fair to say that most people suffer regularly to some degree from a depleted immune system. This sounds like a bold statement, and it is. However, when you look at the factors that are known to depress the system you realise the scale of the problem. Factors that depress immune function include:

stress
poor diet
environmental pollution
lack of exercise
drugs
alcohol
smoking
poor sleeping habits
pesticides, herbicides, preservatives, artificial flavouring and
    colouring agents found in food

How many people do you know who are not affected by one or more of these factors? Virtually everyone in modern society is affected by some item on this list, and the result is wide-scale depression of the immune function.

By far the most devastating of those factors is stress, and sadly, it is the one depressor few modern people can avoid. The mechanism by which stress depresses the immune system is worth our close attention.

When a person is under stress, the pituitary gland produces a hormone called adrenocorticotropin. This hormone floats down to a patch of tissue located on the top of the kidneys and known as the adrenal glands. In response to adrenocorticotropin, the adrenals produce several substances. The first is adrenalin. We are all aware of the adrenalin rush that occurs when we almost have a car crash or nearly fall out of a window. The heart starts beating and the mind races. Adrenalin gets the body moving, and when big things happen, big doses of adrenalin are produced. However, stress causes the production of small amounts of adrenalin. Not enough to make your heart beat faster, but enough to keep you moving through your day. The body was designed to work. Adrenalin is one of the chemicals it produces to keep us alive and moving.

The adrenal glands also produce chemicals known as glucocorticoids at the same time as they produce adrenalin. Glucocorticoids do several things in the body. First, they stimulate the release of sugar into the bloodstream. When you are under stress you need energy to handle whatever situation is causing you stress. The sugar liberated by the glucocorticoids gives you the energy to stay in motion. The second action is a little more sinister: glucocorticoids depress the immune system. They block immune function.

Glucocorticoids are anti-inflammatory. Theoretically speaking, if you are in a fight or flight situation, you might be injured and anti-inflammatory action might be helpful. There is no simple answer other than that this may be a human engineering flaw.

The end result of stress is that the immune system becomes depressed. This is not speculation: it is a statement of fact.

Most of us are aware that stress depresses the immune system. Almost everyone has experienced a major cold after an exam, a big work deadline, a wedding, a divorce, or a death in the family. Many patients have told me that they got sick because they had been stressed out for too long. They may not be aware of the whys and wherefores of the immune system, but they know that being stressed out leaves them vulnerable to infection.

Our lives are spent running—running to catch the bus, to be on time for work, to make the deadline, the evening train, and the evening news. Modern life is incredibly demanding and it is filled with stress. I feel confident in saying that most people have compromised immune systems, because most people have stressful lives. Periods of big stress usually result in a big illness—a bad case of influenza, for example. Moderate stress means a moderate level of immune suppression. There are few who can say they do not suffer from low-grade stress most of the time, and therefore low-grade immune suppression.

This has been a close examination of just one of the factors that depress the immune system. When you add all the other factors to the equation you see how grave the situation has become. When people head into the world every morning they do so without full immunity.

To make matters worse, now is not the time for humans to have a compromised immune system. Now, more than ever, we need fully operational defences. Why is that? First, the modern world is a microbial cesspool. Second, some of the microbes swimming in this cesspool are really bad news. We confront antibiotic-resistant strains of bacteria, strengthened by our very attempt to control them. It's nasty out there, and we are facing this continual attack with weakened forces.

It would pay our whole society to spend more time thinking about microbial pollution (bacteria, virus and fungi). For reasons that elude me, this is a subject that one rarely sees discussed. Whenever you get on a bus or an underground train, you are surrounded by people, people who breathe, cough or sneeze some of their personal populations of microbes into the area around them. When you increase the number of people, you increase the microbial load produced. Public transport has done away with windows in exchange for modern air-conditioning, and in consequence we ride to work in an environment jam-packed with more than commuters. Before we reach the office door we have been bathed and sprayed with microbes. And that is not the end of the story.

The workplace is even worse. My favourite modern phenomenon is what I call the corporate martyr. These long-suffering souls prefer to come in to work sick rather than stay at home where they belong. Indeed, there is some sort of bizarre machismo attached to dragging themselves into the office despite feeling ill. People brag about going in to work sick, and employers actually encourage the behaviour, as if it is doing the world a favour. I think not.

This is really the ultimate act of selfishness. Coming to work, to school, or to play, while sick, puts everyone around you at risk. To make matters even worse, these martyrs work in sealed-air office compounds. As in public transport, windows that open are rare. This means that the air in the office recirculates from floor to floor, and office to office. One corporate martyr can infect hundreds of people in one day with whatever disease he or she is harbouring.

To pursue this theme, let us move on to carcinogenesis, the development of cancer. It is a well established fact that chemicals can cause cells to become cancerous. Workers working with asbestos develop lung cancer because the asbestos fibres cause lung cells to mutate. Pollution (mainly in the form of fossil fuel emissions), food preservatives, pesticides and herbicides—all these are known to cause cancer. The modern world is filled with carcinogens, and it is difficult to avoid these substances. A friend's mother recently died of lung cancer. Neither she nor her husband smoked. She lived in New York City, and walked to work with buses and cars driving alongside her.

The immune system stands between us and cancer on two different levels. First, the immune cells are responsible for picking up carcinogenic matter that makes its way into the body, and getting rid of it before it has a chance to change cells. Failing this, if there are too many chemicals in the body for the immune system to remove, and a few cells become cancerous, it is the immune system's job to kill the cancer cells before they have a chance to grow and spread. To prevent cancer, one needs a functioning immune system on alert, and this is especially true in the modern world. It follows that now would be a great time to have a dynamic immune system.

The solution

Clearly we need to do something to bolster our immune system. Fortunately, like any other system, this can be developed and supported. People who want to can transform themselves from 5-stone weaklings into strapping body-builders by going to the gym five times a week. Many a heart surgery patient has been able to improve his coronary health by changing his lifestyle. Our immune systems may be failing us, but we can do something about it.

On a basic level, the best thing you can do for your immune system is to live a reasonable life. Eat right, sleep right, and take exercise is a good prescription. These three activities will do wonders. The immune system is suspended in the body. Take care of the body, and the immune system will benefit. Many patients say to me: 'Easier said than done.' I ask them to consider the alternative! Failure to support your immune system could result in dire consequences. Cancer and antibiotic-resistant tuberculosis are no walk in the park.

One of the classic Chinese medical texts, *The Yellow Emperor's*

Classic, written in 200 BC, has something that speaks to our present circumstances remarkably. The Yellow Emperor was a real person, and he became concerned when he discovered that his subjects were in poor health and getting worse. These subjects filled his coffers with gold, and the last thing he wanted was for his source of income to be incapacitated. When the Emperor asked his doctors to explain the situation, they responded that the problem with his subjects was their life-style. They had departed from natural living and were paying the price in the form of worsening health. Here is what the Chinese doctors said:

> The men in antiquity lived among their animals. They pursued a vigorous and active life, avoiding in this manner the effects of cold. They sought out shade, thereby avoiding the effects of heat. Their inner life knew no exhaustion from emotions, and their external life was unaffected by the civil service bureaucracy. In that peaceful and satisfied world, evil was unable to penetrate deeply into the body.

The doctors went on to say that though prayer had kept earlier generations healthy, it was not enough in the modern world. For people to stay healthy, they were going to have to do a little more. They were going to have to take medicines. History repeats itself, and medical history is no exception!

We too, the subjects of the Credit Card Emperor, can not rely on maintaining our health by using the old techniques. What once used to work is no longer sufficient. We need to take medicine to stay well. The immune system needs support. This is where immune tonics like *E. angustifolia* fit into the picture. *E. angustifolia* is an agent we can use to counteract the effect of modern living on our body. We need to match weakness with strength. All indicators show that *E. angustifolia* offers us the strength needed to counter our weakness.

The real conclusion
As I said when we began, the journey into *E. angustifolia* is a long haul, not a day-trip. There are all sorts of angles to the

Echinacea story, and as each day passes, the plot thickens. All the same, we are inching, however slowly, towards a better understanding of an amazing medicinal plant, and therefore an ever-widening list of potential applications. If someone studies *E. angustifolia* in cancer, it is possible we may end up with a powerful tool against one of the most lethal human scourges yet to be tamed by the medical world.

As orthodox medicine is now able to cure many of the diseases that formerly took our lives, we have the opportunity to delve into preventive medicine. As the immune system stands between us and most diseases, when you talk about prevention you have to talk about immune tonics. That leads us directly to *E. angustifolia*! Indeed, any substance that stimulates this all-important system is of great interest to the general public, the research and the medical community. It is possible that *E. angustifolia* will become the prototype for a new line of drugs that can revolutionise the world the way penicillin did in the 1940s. The final message from HCR is—watch this space! Now that you have read this book, you have a strong basis to understand what lies ahead as the world of Echinacea unfolds.

Useful Addresses

United Kingdom
General enquiries about finding a practitioner of herbal medicine:

College of Practitioners of Phytotherapy, Bucksteep Manor, Boddle Street Green, near Hailsham, East Sussex BN27 4RG. Tel: 01323 834800.

National Institute of Medical Herbalists, 56 Longbrook Street, Exeter EX4 6AH. Tel: 01392 436022.

General enquiries about herbal medicine and sources of Echinacea:

The Herb Line. Tel: 01323 834800.

Enquiries about the Echinacea species, their use in specific diseases, and sources of additional information:

The Herbalists of Columbia Road (HCR), 140 Columbia Road, London E2 7RG. Tel: 0171 739 9344.

United States
American Herb Guild, PO Box 70, Roosevelt, Utah 84066.
e-mail: ahgoffice@earthline.net

American Botanical Council
www.herbalgram.org

Herb Research Foundation
www.herbs.org

Naturopathic Medicine Network
www.pandamedicine.com

Office of Natural Medicine
altdmed.od.nih.gov

Australia
National Herbalists Association of Australia, Suite 305, 3 Smail Street, Broadway, NSW 2007.

Selected References

Allen, Paul W. *Eclectic System of Medicine*. Published by the Author, New York, 1869.

Barton, William P. C. *Prodrome of a work to aid the teaching of the vegetable materia medica by the natural families of plants in the therapeutic institute of Philadelphia*. 1833.

Bauer, R. and Wagner, H. Echinacea Species as Potential Immunostimulatory Drugs. In: Wagner H., Farnsworth, N. R. (eds.), *Economic and Medicinal Plant Research*, vol. 5. London: Academic Press, 253–321, 1991.

Beach, Wooster. *A Treatise on Anatomy, Physiology, and Health*. Published by the Author, New York, 1847.

Beach, Wooster. *A Medical and Botanical Dictionary*. New York: Baker and Scribner, 1848.

Beach, Wooster. *Beach's Family Physician and Home Guide*. Cincinnati: Moore, Wilstach, and Keys, 1859.

Bruneton, Jean. *Pharmacognosy, Phytochemistry, Medicinal Plants*. Lavoisier, 1995.

Calkins, Marshal. *Thoracic Diseases: Their Pathology, Diagnosis, and Treatment in four parts*. Posthumous writings of Calvin Newton. Philadelphia: Cowperthwait & Company, 1858.

Cox, John Redman. *The American Dispensatory*. Philadelphia: Carey & Lea, 1825.

Densmore, Frances. *Uses of Plants by the Chippewa Indians*. Forty-fifth Annual Report of the Bureau of American Ethnology, 1928.

Duke, James A. *Handbook of Biologically Active Phytochemicals and Their Activities*. Ann Arbor: CRC Press, 1992.

Duke, James A. *Handbook of Phytochemical Constituents of Grass, Herbs and Other Economic Plants*. Ann Arbor: CRC Press, 1992.

Echincaea Purpureae Radix: Purple Coneflower root. First revised version. March 1996. Escop Proposal for the Summary of Product Characteristics.

Ellingwood, Finley. *A Systematic Treatise on Materia Medica and Therapeutics with reference to the most direct action of drugs*. Fifth Edition, thoroughly revised and greatly enlarged. Chicago Medical Times Publishing Company, 1905.

Ellingwood, Finley. *A Manual of the Eclectic Treatment of Disease.* vol. 1. Chicago: Chicago Medical Times Publishing Company, 1906.

Ellingwood, Finley. *A Manual of the Eclectic Treatment of Disease Designed for the Many Students and Practitioners*, in two volumes, vol. 1. Published by the Author, 1907.

Ellingwood, Finley. *American Materia Medica, Therapeutics, and Pharmacognosy.* Ellingwood's Therapeutist. Chicago, 1919.

Felter, Harvey Wickes. *King's Dispensatory*, vols. 1 and 2. Cincinnati: Ohio Valley Company, 1898.

Felter, Harvey Wickes. *Syllabus of Eclectic Materia Medica and Therapeutics.* Compiled from notes taken from the lectures of F. J. Locke, edited with pharmacological additions by H. W. Felter. 2nd ed. with appendix. Cincinnati: Scudder Brothers Company, 1901.

Felter, Harvey Wickes. *History of the Eclectic Medical Institute.* Cincinnati: Eclectic Medical Institute, 1902.

Fyfe, John William. *The Essentials of Modern Materia Medica and Therapeutics.* Cincinnati: The Scudder Brothers Company, 1903.

Fyfe, John William. *Pocket Essentials of Modern Materia Medica and Therapeutics.* Cincinnati: The Scudder Brothers Company, 1911.

Gilmore, Melvin Randolph. *Uses of Plants by the Indians of the Missouri River Region.* 1919.

Gilmore, Melvin Randolph. *A Study in the Ethnobotany of the Omaha Indians.* Collections of the Nebraska State Historical Society. Ed. Albert Watkins. Vol. 17. 1913.

Goss, I. J. M. *The Practice of Medicine on the Specific Art of Healing.* Chicago: W. T. Keener, 1888.

Jones, L. E. and Scudder, J. M. *The American Eclectic Materia Medica and Therapeutics.* Cincinnati: Moore, Wilstach, and Keys, 1858.

King, John. *The American Eclectic Dispensatory.* Cincinnati: Moore, Wilstach, and Keys, 1854.

King, John. *Women: Their diseases and their treatment.* Cincinnati: Longley Brother, 1858

Lloyd, J. U. *Pharmaceutical Preparations: Elixirs.* Cincinnati: Robert Clarke & Company, 1883.

Mundy, William Nelson. *The Eclectic Practice in Diseases of Children for Students and Practitioners.* 2nd ed., revised, rewritten and enlarged. Cincinnati: Scudder Brothers Company, 1908.

Neiderkorn, J. S. *The Physicians and Students Ready Guide to Specific Medication.* Bradford, Ohio: The Little Printing Company, 1892.

Neiderkorn, J. S. *A Handy Reference Book.* Cincinnati: published for the Author, 1905.

Paine, J. *New School Remedies, and Their Application to the Treatment of diseases, including those of Women, Children, and Surgery. Designed for Physicians, Surgeons, Students of Medicine, and Families.* Philadelphia: Claxton, Remsen, & Haffelfinger, 1874

Palmer, Owen. *Diseases of the Digestive Organs for Students and Practitioners of Medicine.* Cleveland, Ohio. 1907.

Peterson, F. J. *Materia Medica and Clinical Therapeutics.* Los Olivos, California: published by the Author, 1905.

Scudder, J. M. *The Eclectic Practice in Disease of Children.* Cincinnati: American Publishing Company, 1869.

Scudder, J. M. *Specific Medication and Specific Medicines.* 5th ed., revised, 1874.

Scudder, J. M. *Specific Diagnosis: A study of Disease with special reference to the administration of Remedies.* Cincinnati: Wilstach, Baldwin, & Company, 1874.

Scudder, J. M. *On the Reproductive Organs and the Venereal.* Cincinnati: Wilstach, Baldwin, & Company, 1874.

Scudder, J. M. *The American Eclectic Materia Medica and Therapeutics.* Cincinnati: published by the Author, 1883.

Scudder, J. M. *The Eclectic Family Physician.* 21st ed., 5th revision. Two vols. in one, with appendix. Cincinnati: John Scudder, 1887.

Scudder, J. M. *A Practical Treatise on the Diseases of Women.* 15th ed., revised. Cincinnati: John M. Scudder, 1891.

Stephens, A. F. *The Essentials of Medical Gynecology. According to the Eclectic, or Specific Practice of Medicine in the Treatment of Disease.* Cincinnati: Scudder Brothers Company, 1907.

Smith, Huron. Ethnobotany of the Meswaki Indians. *Bulletin of the Public Museum of the City of Milwaukee*, vol. 4, no. 2, April 1928.

Towar and Hogan. *The Eclectic and General Dispensatory Comprehending a System of Pharmacy, Materia Medica.* Philadelphia: Mifflin & Parry. 1827.

Thomas, Rolla. *Eclectic Practice of Medicine*, 2nd ed. 1920.

Watkins, Lyman. *An Eclectic Compendium of the Practice of Medicine.* Cincinnati: John M. Scudder's Sons. 1895.

Webster, Herbert T. *The Principles of Medicine as applied to Dynamical Therapeutics.* Oakland, California: published by the Author, 1891.

Webster, Herbert T. *Dynamical Therapeutics—A work devoted to the Theory and Practice of Specific Medication with special references to the newer remedies.* 2nd ed., H. T. Webster, 1898.

Webster, Herbert T. *New Eclectic Medical Practice Designed for Students and Practitioners*, vol. 1. Oakland, California: Webster Medical Publishing Company, 1899.

Webster, Herbert T. *New Eclectic Medical Practice Designed for Students and Practitioners*, vol. 2. Oakland, California: Webster Medical Publishing Company, 1902.